The Middle Distances

Running Seasons and the Wildcats of West Genesee High School

Jim Vermeulen

ISBN 978-1-957077-33-8

Publisher's Cataloging-in-Publication data

Names: Vermeulen, Jim, author.
Title: The middle distances : a running year and the Wildcats of West
Genesee High School / Jim Vermeulen.
Description: Parker, CO: BookCrafters, 2023.
Identifiers: ISBN: 978-1-957077-33-8
Subjects: LCSH West Genesee (N.Y.) | Coaching (Athletics)--Anecdotes.
| Track and field--Anecdotes. | BISAC SPORTS & RECREATION
/ Coaching / General | SPORTS & RECREATION / Track & Field |
SPORTS & RECREATION / Children's & Youth Sports
Classification: LCC GV1060.5 .V47 2023 | DDC 796.4/2--dc23

Publishing assistance by BookCrafters, Parker, Colorado.
www.bookcrafters.net

For Evan,
and the distance runners
of West Genesee High School

"They came and went without announcing they were special."

— James P. Carse

"We try. All of us. We try."

— Richard Ford

The names of most athletes
have been changed for privacy.

Preface

This is a story about runners—high school middle-distance runners to be specific. Over the course of their competitive seasons and their scholastic running years, more than a few of the athletes I coached came to understand, even at a young age, what James Galvin describes as "the recitations of seasons and the repetitive work that seasons require." Their work, of course, is the work of sport in its endless quest for something called excellence. This, then, is a book about the scholastic athletes who sought to master their sport of distance running, never an easy endeavor, and one fully attempted by few. It is not, however, intended to be a traditional sports book. In an age where we have become obsessed with winning and the drama of winners, it is not a book about victors in that typical way of sports stories. Neither of the cross-country teams I coached, boys or girls, overcame all odds or all manner of personal challenges to win the state or national championship in their fall 2019 season. None of my winter indoor or spring outdoor track team members before that became individual state champions. But those who stuck with their sports tried. Some tried harder than others, but most tried in their own way to be successful--and that did matter, regardless of competitive scores or records. This, then, is more a story about what ultimately matters—or should matter--most in high school athletics, which is effort. Effort cannot guarantee excellence; it's not enough. But effort always comes first.

Winter, Spring, Fall--those three running seasons of the 2018/19 school year proved the most trying stretch of my thirty-plus coaching years. I made mistakes, but those mistakes provided some of the best lessons. Dealing with several especially difficult parents, coaching a few athletes who fully believed their eighty percent was a hundred percent—those and other challenges demanded its own type of endurance, but they also reinforced the notion of coaching as the necessary balance of loyalties--loyalty to the athletes, of course, but also loyalty to the sport. Trouble often comes when a coach tips the balance too far one way or the other. Despite all the trials and tribulations, those seasons also reinforced my appreciation that the majority of the athletes who fully embraced this distance running thing got it right--and learned a lot about life. Those athletes, after all, confronted a uniquely difficult test, a fundamental requirement shared with few other athletes in other sports. The degree to which our runners mastered the prolonged and intensifying fatigue that is the heart of distance running simply magnified their individual successes. Their ability to finally appreciate and manage pain was sometimes a mystery to them, but it was also a gift. Our runners, one after the other, learned that nothing truly worthwhile comes cheap.

(February 2023)

Introduction

October 2018 in our part of upstate New York was a month of rain. Or so it seemed. In reality, half of those days were devoid of precipitation or even sunny. But that memory of rain was the product of not my experiencing self, the one which lived that month day by day, hour by hour, but of the remembering self, the one that has the tendency to sum up, to exclude some details and exaggerate others. We had just enough rain-swept days and the muddy mire of a season-ending sectional championship to make the rain, by season's end, seem relentless, which it wasn't.

Both teams had changed significantly from their 2017 predecessors. The girls had lost to graduation two top sectional/state runners, which ended a string of four consecutive state top-25 rankings and one qualification for the state Federation Championship, competitive successes by most measures. Carly and Emily were off to their D1 college teams, leaving behind their considerable talents and a mix of leadership not appreciated until it was gone. The 2017 senior-ladened boys team was less talented than the girls but much more garrulous. On any given day, their presence on the far trails could be triangulated by the loud arguments and laughter of guys who just enjoyed sharing a sport. The trails and back fields had grown quieter once they left.

Re-creating teams was, as typical of high school sports, my primary challenge, but it did not start well when the vital summer mileage preparations of both 2018 squads, voluntary for the athletes, proved lackluster. Only a few achieved their targets, and I was forced to delay much of the harder early-season training to ensure proper base-fitness in the runners—a necessity to avoid injuries. That, of course, constricted their ultimate overall volume of high-quality work and thus their resultant competitiveness as individuals and teams. From the competitive standpoint, neither the boys nor girls teams fared as well as they might have otherwise with proper preparations. Some of the runners were disappointed with those logical consequences. A select few parents were upset, and they looked to blame others. I accepted some of that blame. Honoring a sport is a form of commitment, and fostering commitment, regardless of circumstances, is part of a coach's responsibilities. After the season, I met with the rest of the coaching staff. As we had always counseled our athletes, we objectively critiqued ourselves, we made better plans for the future, and then we moved on.

By conventional wisdom, a Runner's Year begins in June, beneath maximal light. The year counts its way through months and three sports seasons before reaching a climax of fitness and performance roughly eleven months later, the following spring during Outdoor Track. Then, after a few weeks of rest, recuperation and restoration, the cycle repeats itself. Seasons and cycles. For dedicated scholastic distance runners, this pattern conveniently matches the typical school calendar, and so we call it a Running Year.

But that's conventional wisdom. There are some of us who believe that in our part of New York state—the northern part--a runner's identity is measured most distinctly not with the warm beginnings or ends of those cycles, but in the middle, in the dead of winter. The West Genesee school district--and all of central New York--lies east or southeast of Lake Ontario. Typically, northwesterly winds slice down from Canada and search the long fetch of the lake. Much of the winter, Ontario's waters are cold but open. Over its steel-gray surface, westerly winds absorb surface moisture and clouds form. When those clouds bump back across frozen land east and south of the lake, they rise a few hundred feet and snow falls, lots of snow. Lake-effect snow in this part of the country is legendary. When the "indoor" track runners of this region venture outside to train, as they often must, they typically encounter either lake effect snow or the results of that snow. Snowfall makes many of the daily decisions in winter for us. It decides whether school's in or out, whether a scheduled meet is on or cancelled, whether it's possible to accomplish anything practical with an outdoor practice. In upstate, we have in no way weather-proofed our winter sport. The weather, instead, sculpts us. Weather is not some abstract dimension of the runners' sport during those cold months. On more days than they wish, working the weather is a major element of their sport. To really understand dedicated upstate scholastic middle-distance runners, you look for them first in winter.

Winter

"You gotta be going there to get there."
— Anonymous

The crows were on the move too. Near dusk, high above a clump of runners tracing back roads through light snow, the crows slid like black dots across a white erase-board. They were arcing toward a neighboring upstate city and any residual heat they hoped to find for the night. As light began to fade, the temperature fell. Snowfall was building.

Below, the runners picked up their paces. They knew they would reach the bright warmth of the high school before car headlights came on. They were assured of their final destinations and their comforts of the evening, so they cinched up parka collars and elbowed themselves into the wind.

And the crows flapped on, driven to expect far less.

November

***

Athletes:

You are receiving this e-mail because you have either signed up for indoor track or attended our pre-season meeting with the intention of doing so.

Welcome to Wildcats Indoor Track. Welcome to our cramped, third-of-the-upper-gym 'home.' Welcome to our tight-cornered, stuffy hallways. Welcome to stairwells that double as plyometric stations. Welcome to our cold macadam parking lots, usually cleared of snow but not always of cars. Welcome to our neighborhood roads where we race the early-season darkness, where we jog to the long tilt of 'The Rise' that sometimes accommodates our total-team "happy family" workouts. And welcome to our Monte Vista hill that climbs an old drumlin and will challenge you, whether in late November t-shirts or geared up for February 20o up-and-around half-mile intervals. Welcome to the long winter weeks and the all-around-the-place 'messiness' that is Indoor Track.

Does it all sound like difficulties and discouragements? Hardly. You never had it so good.

You might not know this, but a few decades ago, the sport you've just joined did not exist in our district. For expediency, and as a sop to the community that had voted down the school budget, a former superintendent recommended to the Board of Education that Indoor Track be cut. The board agreed, and your district became the only large school in the area without a program. In your time span, of course, that's all ancient history, but what shouldn't be dismissed is that parents and coaches and athletes way back then fought hard to reinstate the sport, though it took eleven years. And when they finally succeeded, appreciative athletes worked even harder to honor the opportunity to practice and compete. They held team meetings in a hallway where rain and meltwater seeped in. They ran hurdles on hard tiles. They hopped one-legged up dimly lit stairwells. By our second year back, we were up to thirty team members, and four of them went to the state championship.

A lot has happened since those early seasons. Our team sizes, with some fluctuations, have grown. We survived several refugee years after a ridiculous hallway-use prohibition banished us to practice two seasons in the chilly, dimly lit buildings of the NYS Fairground--and then another winter scratching frozen condensation from cold bus windows on our way home from workouts at a local indoor soccer facility. Nobody complained. The athletes managed to have fun and make adversity an ally.

Along the way, we've had sectional champions, state championship medalists. We've had state and Federation champions. We've even had national All-Americans and grade-level national champions. But for all those talented athletes, we've had many more with highly successful seasons, not because they won leagues or 'went states,' but because they committed to mastering an event through hard work and personal sacrifice in pursuit of a worthy athletic goal. They set the standards. They paved your way. Those are the former athletes— your predecessors—you should quietly thank the next time you have the chance to muscle the apex of a sharp hallway turn or cinch up the hood and head out into the snow for a neighborhood run on the roads.

We've never been one of the so-called "popular" sports. And that doesn't really matter. What matters is whether indoor is popular to *you*, because you are the sport's most important constituent. Your predecessors proved it was popular to them--repeatedly. There's an old saying: "wind extinguishes a candle but energizes a fire." Aside from the very literal fact you'll be dealing with some stiff winds this winter on The Rise or up Monte Vista hill, what the saying recommends is that you come into the season burning with the desire and the determination to excel personally. If you do, our training (that would be the wind) will ignite your true potential as an athlete. Then you'll be personally accomplished, a valuable contributor to the team, and feel pretty good about yourself as a result.

I've been around awhile. I understand and appreciate the standards of effort and excellence set by your alumni predecessors. The fitness trainer of the Uruguayan national soccer team used to tell his athletes, "The effort is not negotiable." That was true for former team members, and it remains true for you. Talent is talent, but ultimately, it's effort by which you will more often be judged—and rewarded.

Come into the season prepared. Come ready to be challenged, both physically and mentally. The expectation to "be better than yourself" will be daily, but that's why you do sports. One of my father's favorites (and one he passed on too often) is that "if it's worth doing, it's worth doing well." Expect to do this season well.

So welcome to Wildcat Indoor Track. We start next Monday, November 19th. Show up on Day 1 ready to work. See you then.

—Coach Vermeulen

***

I woke up to snow on the ground and snow falling. *Bring it on*, was the thought, even though I knew this early light blanket in mid-November could vanish just as quickly as it came and that we might, before Christmas, conduct a few Indoor Track practices in sixty-degree T-shirt weather. Still, more of the white stuff was forecast in the form of an ominous coastal system, one that had meet planners on edge for Saturday's NYS Cross-Country Federation Championship in Poughkeepsie. Usually, I would have shared their concern, but for the first time in a number of years, my teams had neither individual nor team qualifiers for that championship. I had been reduced to a mere, and distant, spectator. That typical overlap of the cross-country and indoor track seasons had always been more a reinforcement—and never the curse—of coaching distance runners. This year, though, I had a few days off. As that beast storm crawled northward, I could easily imagine 3-4 months of steel-cold Indoor Track weather ahead. The cross-country chapter was behind me. Snow had turned the page.

***

Going into a season, as a coach you are granted that fleeting luxury of anticipation. You are allowed your fleeting fantasies before the eventual realities come crashing down. Making reasoned predictions about the season ahead, then, usually hinges on tempering imagined possibilities with the concrete past. And even then, most would argue that, with adolescent athletes, the past cannot with any certainty be considered prelude to the future. Their volatile lives change too quickly. Still, with most seasons, many of the names on the roster are familiar—and that provides a reasonable indication of what's to come. That familiarity means, for me, a recorded history of workout data, performance marks, casual observations, and stories. Of the veterans, I know all the personal records and all the workout results season to season, year to year because I keep a lot of records. I also know who tends to 'come up big' in the championships and who is prone to faltering, who's a competition workhorse at meets with multiple events and who's a one-and-done'er. My database history of rosters also reveals if an athlete has committed to the long haul--that steady accumulation of miles and seasons that indicates investment--or simply dabbles in the sport with a season here, a season there. Those archived facts of an athlete's running life are on my flash drive for handy retrieval.

But it's the stories—some of them short--you can tell yourself about this or that person which really matter most. So-and-so was battling a bad head cold at one afternoon practice and could have begged off the day but didn't, gutting out the intervals instead.

[14]

Another who was asked during a competitive meet to add a second event when a teammate fell ill and, without batting an eye, nodded and said, "I can do that coach." Or even another who could be seen with an arm wrapped around a neophyte's shoulders following that newbie's disastrous race, offering support in a low whisper. I know I can create pages of 'data' about any athlete when considering his or her potential for the season ahead. I have all those records. But if asked to make predictions about a particular someone, what I often come back to are the stories.

***

Our average-sized group assembled on the gym floor for Day 1 of Indoor Track team practices struck various poses. The casual reclines of the veterans contrasted with the wide-eyed forward leans of newbies attentive to their first taste of varsity participation. They didn't want to miss a thing.

Opening days are like snowflakes. They look familiar but always present a unique patina of intrigue. They always come with questions. How many of the on-line sign-up roster will actually show? Will those 'sure thing' athletes actually be the sure things this season? And then you can bank on some of the drama that only young adults manage to pull off. A few years ago, a young lady huffed up to me after attendance on a first day. "You didn't call my name," she indignantly informed me.

Hands on hips, she announced that name, and I checked. "Well, Stacy," I told her, "that would be because you are not on the roster." I showed her the on-line list that, minus her moniker, had been updated one last time only the previous hour.

Completely nonplussed--and with a trace of irritation--Stacy declared, "My mother was supposed to sign me up."

"Yes, well, apparently she didn't," I told her. "But you can stay and watch practice if you'd like."

With no Stacy this year, and against a backdrop of bouncing basketballs from the boys varsity practice in our other two-thirds of the upstairs main gym, attendance went smoothly. Several of the called names were met with silence, and eventually a voice would

[16]

waft from the back of the group: "he's not doing it." These MIA's, typically 10% on Day 1, had been a constant over the years, either students with second thoughts or, sometimes, those who'd signed up on a lark, never intending to ever don shorts and training shoes.

With lines squiggled through those phantoms on the attendance sheet, it was time for The Speech. My first-day speeches had always been remarkably unspectacular, nothing that would ever cut it in a football pre-game locker room. Practice and preparation improved their content but never their delivery, so the best tactic was to shorten them, something the athletes, if polled, would heartily endorse. I delivered the usual "we have a lot of talent on both teams," because that was, in fact, true. Ours was ten straight years of eventually sending boys or girls athletes to the state championship, and now with Dan, Jake, Easais and Pat, four fast and motivated senior sprinters, year eleven looked a distinct possibility. I segued quickly into the heart of the matter with a no-cut team, which wasn't raw talent. Effort, I told them, was a personal attribute not dependent on athleticism, so they'd be judged primarily by their daily efforts. And, I added with a nod, you can't make efforts if you don't show up. "You are expected to make a commitment to the season and what the sport requires" was the summation. No one jumped to their feet afterward, hooting and applauding wildly.

Our first-day concerns had taken extra time, so after a hallway warm-up and drills, the entire team was reassembled outside on the school's lower parking lot. Snow still covered the track, and the days were still shortening. Because we had a fair number of newbies, both my assistant, Coach Palmisano, and I wanted to keep them close. We wanted to watch together and compare notes. Early on in any season, whether it's during a warm-up, movement drills or the runs of a practice, you learn the most just by watching. Athletes, though they seldom realize it, simply announce themselves through gestures and behaviors. They think they're invisible while safely nestled in their groups, but if you're watching, if you're paying attention and know what you are looking for, they are anything but. Certain challenges, like listening to directions, were already apparent. Most of the enthusiastic group were appropriately dressed in layers--and some also wore hats and gloves. A few, despite my previous gear e-mails and suggestions at our pre-season meeting, shivered in their T-shirts and shorts.

The afternoon was typical for late November—cloudy, cool, gray to a fault, but calm. We'd strategically placed orange cones to warn any entering cars of the runners sharing their space. For good measure, I stood with our volunteer coach, Tim, at the entrance from the old upper circle, directing the occasional car to either wait or veer left into a far empty corner of the lot. The team members circled, running a minute and a half at General Conditioning pace, or about 70% of all-out effort. Then, on Coach P's whistle, they would surge and run thirty to forty seconds at their 'up' pace. Coach had announced that intensity as 85%. Unfamiliar with his metric, I told my veteran distance runners it was more like their strong threshold paces.

In the still, chilly air, it took only a few minutes for the physical sorting to begin. Clumps of runners formed, stretched, then broke into smaller clumps. Some in those groups pumped their arms too vigorously, some clomped down on heels or wagged shoulders side to side, all a mechanical confirmation that efficient running is not necessarily natural; it's a skill that sometimes needs improving. Others just gunned their ups, then groaned, unfamiliar or inadept at measuring out the effort, pacing the work. The shot put and weight throwers, in general, weren't having fun, but I'd warned them earlier that over the course of the season they would certainly be running too. Others weaved around them as though navigating agility cones. A few of our new self-designated sprinters ran out of gas after only a few minutes, their ups becoming less and less distinguishable from their downs. And several neophyte middle-distance hopefuls initially tagged along with our veterans but soon began to 'fall off the wagon' as enthusiasm confronted fatigue. Most of the veterans went calmly about the business of Day 1, which was unglamorous. They had been there before. To the rest, I muttered quietly, *Welcome to Indoor Track.*

Around and around they paced. Coach blew the whistle and they slowed. Coach blew the whistle again and most of them managed to surge. A car meandered in, stopped, and some students peered out its front window with looks of amused pity. Around and around. The muted afternoon daylight ebbed further. Coach blew his whistle one last time and they shuffled to a stop, relieved but apprehensive. It was only the end of their first set.

***

The afternoon sky was dull with clouds that sealed us beneath them like an overturned bowl. Up the steep rise of Monte Vista hill, the dark macadam lay spotted with the white smears of salt-melt left from the weekend's storm. Our sprinters pushed their intervals up one side of the street, then descended in slow trudges down the other. Coach P. was keeping them to that short, steep section. My distance runners were following the fast-twitchers at a slower pace, but then continuing up and around the .4 mile loop that circles the drumlin's flat apex, an isolated terrain where houses seem to float above the neighborhood below. A tiny rip in the clouds momentarily teased the athletes with splotches of sun—and then the afternoon darkened again.

Layered up in warm clothes, Coach P. stood halfway up the hill, monitoring his sprinters, edging them further off to the side whenever the occasional car climbed past or descended. I stayed atop the hill, cajoling or complimenting the distance runners—whichever worked best—as they labored their up and arounds. The day's gloom was eased by a lack of wind. It was another of those listless, overcast late November afternoons that, but for the athletes' heavy breathing, was shrouded in silence.

Up the hill and headed into her fourth long interval plugged Terri, a team neophyte who'd agreed to try the distance group for a week and was now probably wondering what the hell she'd gotten into. As she plugged doggedly by, the sky drained to a deeper gray.

***

I stopped Cindy and Pam on their hallway warm-up just to let Cindy know it would improve her form if she relaxed the arms a little and drove the elbows back further with each stride. She was running with tightly clinched arms and hunched shoulders, as though trying to inch her way through a bunched subway crowd. It's a common misconception that all new young runners are naturals with body movement. Sometimes they are not. Some have developed their own habits, which can be bad ones. Often, effective running mechanics have to be taught, and sometimes inefficient movements have to be un-taught first. Watch a new runner with arms tucked up too tight like Cindy's, and it's a safe bet you're looking at a soccer player who's been tutored in that defensive posture for warding off opponents. I quickly showed Cindy how to relax the arms and to check with peripheral vision for proper elbow drive that brings hands brought back close to the body mid-line. "It'll make you more efficient and faster," I told her.

Cindy took the opportunity to ask, "Are we going outside today?" Beyond the large plate glass windows of the hallway, it was snowing steadily, but lightly, and snowmelt was already visible as expanding wet spots.

"Yup," I told her, you're outside."

"But I don't want to go outside," she protested, though with a wry smile. I laughed, pulled out my air-violin and started playing sad, phantom notes. With good-natured scowls, she and Pam took off down the hall to rejoin their group. When they came back around, I was still playing.

Laura

In early December, with the rest of her teammates already weeks into their winter sports at the high school, Laura was leaving singular tracks in the morning frost that coated our cross-country training trails at Camillus Middle School. Less than a week from then, she would trade northeast chill for the heat and dust of San Diego's Balboa Park and the Footlocker National Championship. Sophomore Laura had pushed the pace hard at her state and NY Federation cross-country championships, leading late in those races only to be caught and passed by others at the end. Stubbornly resolute, she employed the same tactic at the Footlocker Northeast Regional Qualifier--leading halfway at Long Island's Sunken Meadows Park 5k before coming undone on steep and sandy "Cardiac Hill." Through sheer will, she rallied late in the race, and a 5th place finish had punched her ticket to the national championship. After her frigid preparatory work-out, with a weak sun straining to melt out evidence of her passages, I quickly reviewed that November string of front-runner gambles. Then I asked, "So, how's that race strategy working for you?" Laura mumbled and grumbled, then she flew to San Diego a week later, where she employed a brilliantly executed wait-and-surge tactic to finish third in the nation.

Following a transitional rest period, Laura plunged into winter track, heart set on qualifying to race the Millrose Games high school Invitational Mile in February. The best of the best. The first months went well; she pushed herself hard, and late in January toed the New Balance Invitational start line at New York City's Armory Track & Field Center. The two final qualifying spots for Millrose were up for grabs. Positioning herself safely, Laura let the race favorites work the lead into the final two laps. Then she powered around a Virginia runner and eyed the substantial twenty-meter gap to the now-presumed winner, yet another resident of the Old Dominion state. With another lap, that gap had shrunk to ten meters, and down the back stretch of the bell lap, Laura closed to the leader's shoulder. She didn't wait, but geared down and passed on the turn, then fought off her competitor along the final meters to win a spot at the Millrose Games. Hers was also a new a Section III indoor mile record. Three days later, after the doctor had confirmed a metatarsal stress fracture, the Millrose Games and Laura's indoor season simply vanished.

Stress fractures heal slowly. Outdoor Track that spring was a series of fits and starts, light training and high hopes dashed repeatedly by setbacks.

The season passed her by. Everyone hoped a summer of good training would lead to a strong junior-year rebound. It did—and it didn't. There was a failure to qualify for a second Footlocker Nationals, but during Indoor Track, Laura made it back to Millrose and placed 3rd. She won her second Loucks Games 2000 meter Steeplechase in the spring, but then missed All-American in that event at nationals, finishing 8th. Throughout, the foot never seemed totally right. Her parents even drove her to Virginia and a specialized gait-analysis lab. Laura came home with an impressive DVD of foot-strikes and body angles but no satisfying solutions. In her final senior cross-country season, she had the lowest State and Federation championship finishes of her high school career.

Laura's final Indoor Track season came with its requisite cold, snowy roads and hard-tiled high school hallways. She hung tough in December, completing good workouts and slowly improving her races. I caught the occasional guarded smile. In early January, she failed at a first attempt to qualify again for Millrose but a few days later lined up for the 3000 meter race at our section's Constantino Invitational. Alongside were two talented Fayetteville-Manlius competitors, both who had raced in December on their national champion cross-country team. For the first nine laps of fifteen, they formed a tight trio. Then Laura dialed up a strong tenth lap and pulled away. There were still five laps to go, but the body language and turn-over of her competitors signaled the race for first was over.

After, I walked up to congratulate her on the win and a school record in that event. Self-demanding and sometimes taciturn to the point of speechlessness, all Laura ever really wanted was to be able to train hard and race even harder. Bent over, hands on knees, she twisted her face upward between breaths, smiled quickly and gasped, "That felt sooo good!"

December

I was early to the high school for our meet departure, the first contest of the season. Some of the athletes had been absent for the earlier handouts of our school competition singlets and shorts, so I lugged those out again and set myself in the hallway by the locker rooms. I snagged my customers as they wandered in.

When Tammi stepped up to claim her shorts, on a thought I shooed the others away. Coach P. walked up, but when I motioned to hold off for moment, he instantly recognized and backed off. Tammi stared down at me. "Tammi," I said quietly in our little zone of privacy, "Are there any adults in your life who you really trust?"

This wasn't just some curious, inappropriate question plucked from nowhere and for no good reason. Only the day before, as we prepared for team drills, two of her teammates had approached to say Tammi was in a hallway bathroom, crying. And three days earlier than that, Tammi had missed both school and practice for what her father informed me were "family issues." Beyond that, backward stretched many other difficult weeks, seasons, and even a team suspension for a school athletic policy infraction. But we'd always kept the door open, and Tammi had always hung on. She'd known instinctively that the days were typically better with sports and her teammates.

Tammi seemed a little surprised by the question, but she gave it some thought. "My mom," she said, smiling as though just reminded of a fond memory. "I can talk to her about anything."

"Well that's good," I told her. "That's good." Then I related the story of ringing the doorbell at the home of a former runner who was extremely talented but navigating a tortured family life. I was at that runner's house, I told Tammi, late after another practice afternoon he had missed. I went to talk him out of quitting track because I knew that, despite all the turmoil, this sport and his sports buddies could probably be the best part of his day, a port in the storm. I didn't want him to add that failure to all his other losses. "I'm not saying it's the same at home for you, Tammi. I'm just saying that being on the team, being with your buddies—that is the same positive. So I hope it helps."

Tammi smiled. We talked a little about her sudden episodes of crying. No, she didn't know what caused them, she said they just happened. But with friends around, they would pass. "Well," I told her. "I hope things get better. Are you O.K. for today?" She shook her head yes and wandered off to the locker room. The other athletes pressed in, anxious for their shorts and singlets. They had a team bus to catch.

***

Monday. It was another Grunt Monday. The middle-distance squad, alone this afternoon because throwers were training with sprinters in the school's upper hallways, jogged in small groups through the neighborhood toward a Monte Vista Drive afternoon. They trotted and gabbed beneath our typical shrouded sky, late Fall steadily fading toward the coming harshness of winter. The runners had three sets of three long intervals on the agenda, those four-tenths of a mile up-and-arounds. To enhance muscle recruitment, we sometimes finish each set with a "blaster," a full sprint up the initial steep of the circuit. But not that day. Through experience, their Monday workouts work best without required precision or raw speed. What they demand, however, is raw effort and persistence, a put-your-head-down-and-go kind of day. A Grunt Monday. Our runners had grown to appreciate the concept.

I parked the car near the base of the hill and opened the back for any extra layers the runners wanted to shed and store. Instructions only took a moment because most were veterans of the workout. They milled, grouped, crossed Forsythe Street to the start at the base of the Monte Vista hill. Then, with deep breaths and leaning shoulders, they set out. I walked up the hill and took my place at the top of the steep rise. From there, the runners would be lost to sight for a short time as they circled the top loop before curving back at me and the finish. Their full circuits formed a dyslexic "p" with most of the distance hung in the sky atop our isolated drumlin.

The day quickly fell into a workmanlike rhythm, and any passersby could be forgiven for mistakenly concluding only a repetitious drudgery, efforts absent the excitement of a three-point basketball shot from a deep corner or a curving soccer kick just beyond the leaping stretch of a goalie into the net's upper right corner. It's hard to explain the satisfaction of the grind, holding a pace over a series of increasingly exhausting intervals. It's difficult to quantify the personal rewards of summoning muscle contractions to actually finish faster. Many of the daily victories are private and resistant to description, exertions that prompt blank expressions later at home when the question comes up, "how was practice today?"

Another question that resists easy answers is the one of what effect recent performances will have on these young adults once back at training. We were now two days beyond Saturday's Morse Relays, time enough for the heightened emotions—whatever they were—to settle and allow the competitive air to clear. Practical wisdom dictates that coaches show patience with après-race discussions or analytics. Earnest in-your-face do-and-don't harangues just beyond the finish line may feel timely—and they may look from afar like passionate coaching--but they are often just a useless stirring of the existing stew of strong emotions. For good reasons, the coaching elders preach a 24 hour wait rule.

Both teams had finished 8th, well back in the 12-team pack. Typically, the majority of our athletes were just getting their feet wet in that first meet. 'Shaking off the rust' is another popular misnomer. Wide eyes on the neophytes combine with the dogged winces of veterans, all confronting just how much preciseness or sustained quickness their events demand. Going into the seasons, we always tell the athletes that track done right is hard, and those first meets always manage to drive the point home. Terri had run an anchor 800 meter in the JV sprint medley relay, her first track event ever, and in lap three of four, she hit the wall hard, struggling the last two hundred meters to the finish. I gave her that welcome-to-indoor-track look coupled with a wry smile and a quick pat on the shoulder. No smile came back, but I knew she'd be alright. It was Tammi who had me wondering. Her 800meter leg in the 4x800 was lukewarm, nothing personally great, certainly nothing tragic, an effort that appeared mostly time put in, a chore completed, like cleaning up your room. She had, at least, raced the 2nd fastest split of her relay group which finished second, the team's best competitive result of the meet. I had simply told the squad that theirs was a good enough start to the season, which it was, and I turned to other events. First meets, though, also produce some head-scratchers, so when I walked over to the line official and told him to DQ our just-finished boys 4x800 because my #2 guy had only run three of his required four laps, he just shook his head and smiled.

A few of the runners on Sunday had submitted their voluntary Race Analysis's. We keep them brief and voluntary, short recapitulations of their perceived strengths and weakness of competitive efforts--and any of their plans for improvement. They are guaranteed my reply.

Terri returned hers, considering a strength "not giving out," noting a weakness of not pacing properly and hoping to improve that in the future. I sensed a Freudian slip. "I assume," was my reply, "that you mean, 'Not giving up.'" Then I advised her to take advantage of all practice opportunities to improve her basic foot speed and look to train with faster team members. "Be patient," I wrote, "but persistent. Especially in distance running, good things take time." Tammi was less definitive with her analysis, writing that she was "unsure" of any strengths but that her weakness was "Mental strength, pushing myself harder." She wanted "to be able to push myself harder and calm my nerves more before races."

The afternoon light of Monte Vista Drive waned as the runners accumulated intervals and fatigue. Some were destined to complete only two of the planned three sets of work, enough for their days. Sara and Cindy had paired for the workout, and as I watched Cindy struggle to stay with Sara on the up-and-around, I wondered if her 1500 meter disappointment at that first meet—one that brought tears—was merely being compounded. But she rallied, keeping pace up the steep and not falling too far off her teammate around the top oval. After, I pulled her aside and asked, "Do you know what persistence means?" She shot me a dismissive of course look, so I just patted her on the shoulder. "Well, that's all you need."

Pam and Tammi were two of the last runners off the hill. In the gathering gloom, they charged their final finish, the fastest of the girls' efforts that afternoon. I congratulated them on a job well done. We stood at the top of the steep for a moment as they gathered themselves with deep breaths. Then Tammi asked, "Do you remember you said we could talk if I wanted." Of course, I told her, and after she quickly glanced at Pam she said, "Then can we talk?" I looked at the runners below us, now off the hill and small with distance, writing times on the practice sheet at my car before starting their jog back to the high school. "I mean, we could talk later if you want," Tammi hurriedly added. "No," I told her, "this is fine. Do you mind if Pam's with us?"

Pam, of course, was exactly the person Tammi wanted with her. The three of us stood in the cool grey afternoon as two final runners descended the hill. Tammi described her uncertainties about the indoor track season. She did not feel she could put her heart into the practices. She was unhappy with a desultory effort in Saturday's 4x800 relay. I reminded both of them how early it was in the season, how improvements would come. "I can't explain it," Tammi said, as though I was missing her point. "I don't know the word."

I was fairly sure I did. "I think the bigger issue," I told her, "is that you're wondering if you still love the running enough, that you still have the passion for it. Right?" Tammi shook her head yes. We talked some more. Tammi described feeling responsible for--or loyal to--what her parents wanted, to what her teammates wanted, to what I wanted. The grey afternoon around us had gone quiet. With Pam listening and quietly nodding, I told Tammi that all those people she mentioned cared about her. I said she was a good teammate and it would be a less enjoyable team without her, but that the decision about participating ultimately belonged to her. The last thing I suggested was that she talk with her parents again. I made no promises but reminded her that the program and her teammates and the coaches would always be there.

She and Pam jogged slowly down the hill, logged their third set time on the practice sheet and were off toward the high school before I even reached the car. I drove back through dusk. Car headlights along West Genesee Street had come on. Later, after core drills in our gym space, I pulled Pam aside before she left and asked what she thought Tammi wanted to do. Pam looked at me and said, "She wants to quit."

***

Our 'Field Events' practice day seemed to click. Outside, the temperature had steadied itself in the low 20's, and the light snow that had fallen most of the day retreated, leaving only a dull gray blanket of clouds. The distance runners headed out into that on a fartlek run, but other team members stayed inside to work the jumps and throws and to hone hurdle technique.

Field Event days highlight the inherent renegade nature of Indoor Track programs. Most teams have their tidy rectangular practice areas—the basketball and volleyball courts, the pool, the wrestling room. An indoor team, most days, simply scatters, with some outside running the roads, some plying the hallways or lifting in the weight-room, and others crammed into some found space for long jump or high jump or pole vault training. Normally, this athletic diaspora functions smoothly, but there are those afternoons when the scattered activity can seem just this side of manageable mayhem, with coaches trying to make sure everyone is in the right place at the right time and doing the right thing. Most of the teacher, administrator or community complaints about our Indoor athletes come when athletes wander off with ideas of their own. We have a carefully crafted sentence in our Team Handbook that emphasizes the responsibility required of team members when dispersed. And we lean heavily on that requirement— but these are teenagers, after all. They are not above occasionally testing the rules.

The day was somewhere in between. With my distance runners organized for their run outdoors, then 'stick drills' in the hallway to improve turnover, and finally Weight Room work with Coach Mosotti, the school's strength consultant, I found myself at one point in the upper gym with hurdlers, throwers, high jumpers and long/triple jump athletes—all trying to squeeze in practice time. Tim, our volunteer coach, needed to leave early, and Coach P. was in the upstairs hallways with non-field event sprinters. Fortunately, our main gym was empty, set up for a 5:00 p.m. junior varsity basketball game, so we had all of it until 4:30 sharp, courtesy of a deal I'd struck with the custodians who would need to Zamboni the court and power out the motorized stands in time. We had just time enough.

I watched Dave, short-legged Dave, who had no business training so hard with the high hurdle event except for a desire to help the team. He was tutoring Karen on trail-leg technique. Tara and I, with a few others, were working on high jump. Tara had other favored events and was not particularly fond of high jumping but had agreed to my deal, which was to train and compete only occasionally until the championships when we'd need her athleticism and high jump team points. Jerry was up at the far end of our improvised long and triple jump runway, the one that ended in two mats braced against the retracted south bleachers. He was helping several teammates set their runway marks. One of those was Sandy. Sandy was a neophyte experiment, but given her sprint speed, the event was worth a shot. Long jump might work for her; it might not. We would never know unless she tried.

Off my right shoulder, close enough for me to instruct both them and jumpers, the throwers were finishing up drills and starting shot put and weight throws into another set of old mats against the west wall. Coach Corley, our outdoor track throws specialist, had worked briefly with them the previous day, and they were now implementing his corrections.

The high windows of the gym had grown dark with the approaching winter solstice, but in the bright glare of the gym lights, our groups were busy, filling the place with shouts and friendly razzings for poorly executed technique. If I watched closely enough and compared what I was seeing with memories of previous field events practices, I could identify some of those pleasant improvements by athletes who had been diligent with their training time. And it does take time. The German writer, Johann Goethe, addressed the obvious: "Everything is hard before it is easy." The moment when something becomes 'easy' for an athlete, though, is the surprise that's not really a surprise. And the process toward 'easy' always illuminates. Watching an athlete going through the 'hard' parts tells you a lot about that soon-to-be adult.

Coach Palmisano eventually came down from the upper halls with his non-field event sprinters. The distance runners had returned, finished their 'sticks' and Weight Room work and were shouldering packs to head out. Coach and I sat for a moment after practice, watching custodians extend the stands and ready the scorers' table for the 5:00 p.m. game. "How'd it go?" he asked. I reached for a mental inventory of the afternoon but came up short. Game spectators began trickling in at the far end of the gym. I stood up to pull on my coat. "I think it went O.K.," I finally told him. "No, it went pretty well."

The email came in 5:36 a.m. on Wednesday, the week before our holiday break.

Coach, I won't be able to come to practice until after January 9 because I am going on vacation today.
Jason

Jason:

Thank you for contacting me. Your current team attendance is 52%. If you returned on January 9th, your attendance at that point would be 33%. I appreciate you were honest enough to inform me you missed our 12/15 team bus for the Jensen Invitational because you overslept. That missed meet, plus the earlier missed 12/8 first invitational due to a lack of state-required practices, plus the two meets you will miss due to your family vacation and your subsequent 33% attendance means you could not obtain the team-required attendance to qualify for the 1/11 or 1/19 meets. You are not meeting our attendance guidelines. You are not "showing up," the basic requirement for every team member. Unfortunately, I must remove you from the team roster. Please return your school singlet to me through a teammate.

Jason, during Indoor Track 2017-18, you stopped coming to practices in mid-January and then you left that team. You are talented and could be a strong, contributing teammate, but showing up comes first. If you decide to compete on future indoor or outdoor track teams, please understand that attendance and effort will always be required.

Good luck with the rest of your school year,
Coach Vermeulen

Later that morning, I forwarded the email exchange to Coach Palmisano. An hour later, he got back to me: "Enough is enough."

***

The temperature had soared, hitting a record 65° by 2 p.m. T-shirts and shorts greeted the first day of winter. Coach P. was grumbling about the effectiveness of his pre-meet day routine. He considered whether it needed to be more demanding, more precise. I told him I had no problem with either—or both for that matter--providing the athletes did not show up at the meet arena the next day 'flat' or tired. The middle-distance crew was sent on a 20-minute general conditioning run, then returned for strides and sprints. I pulled together Saturday's 4x400 girls squad, which included two distance runners, for baton drills. After the prolonged fatigue of their other races, our distance runners usually considered racing the 4x400 a treat. Where some of the sprinters expressed displeasure at the notion of 'extending' their range up to 400 meters, for distance runners, stepping down and going full tilt for just two laps of the indoor track had always been a blast. And our best middle-distance runners, as history attests, had usually been good at it. On our 16/17 and 17/18 4x400 girls relays--each which medaled at the state championship—both of those squads included three middle-distance runners.

This group was different. The prospect of two quick laps seemed to weigh on them. And I was getting frustrated with Sara—again. Talented, she had a desultory approach to just about anything we did, and she often signaled, with her look-away gaze, that most training information or suggestions were of little interest. Another coach had suggested that, because of her natural athleticism, things had always come too easily to her. He thought that the notion of working hard for small corrections and improvement was foreign to her, never worth the effort. I had my own theory. It was that the sport was not her favorite and had been someone else's choice. Proxy expectations are always poor substitutes for personal initiative and investment. Whatever the cause, the irritation in my voice about her sloppy body position and half-hearted arm extension for the handoff must have been apparent. But it wasn't helping matters. So, I took a breath to relax, and tried again.

***

The short of it was that many of the team members continued to improve. If Coach P. and I were doing our jobs, of course, that was the expectation. At the Saturday Constantino Invitational, our third competition, the girls' team produced their best collective effort, finishing 5th in the 17-team field, a half point out of 4th. One of our stronger runners had left early for the vacation break. Her absence had cost them that higher place finish, but I doubt anyone but myself and Coach P. were aware of that consequence. The boys placed 8th, matching their Morse finish, but, like the girls, one of their most talented members was also missing. In the boys' tightly packed field, that absence was a loss of two places for the team. Coach and I kept those lost opportunities to ourselves.

In the boys 1600 meter, I had watched Matt charge out enthusiastically and shadow the leaders. Lap times slowed in the middle, where expected, but he pushed on and finished strong, with a personal record, third place, and his first Indoor sub 4:40 the result. Despite that, he had struggled late in the race with stronger competitors using their superior upper body strength to muscle ahead of him. More future time in the weight room was the solution, but I saved the speech. I remembered an athlete who, years before, had set a personal record. After being informed of possible improvements, he took me to task with a good-natured smile and shake of the head. "You're never satisfied." Instead, I simply congratulated Matt. I was learning. He then added a 4th in the 1000 meter, so his was a good day, a solid double. Later, he would e-mail his Race Analysis:

[39]

I'll do the 3200m and the 1600m. I like the pressure of another event soon to come. I also think it's good training. Hoping to get the state time in the 1600m and drop under 10min for the 3200m. If I do this, then I can focus on the 1000 and getting the state time for that. I want to prove that I improved, not just by numbers but mentally as well. As soon as my hip is healed, I can focus on keeping it heathy and training consistently. I should be able to achieve my goals with just a little patience.

The job is straightforward, though usually difficult. You build the runner to the point where performance makes a good match with enthusiasm.

Standing near the start line and clicking lap times, I watched Pam take fourth in the 1500m, meeting the sectional championship standard and later racing a solid leg in the 4x400 relay, suggesting the future. I imagined her making the state championship in a year or two. I watched Cindy run a wide-eyed 1000 meter race, bumping into a realization that this distance running thing is hard. That big question still lay on her horizon, but it was coming closer: is this worth it? I watched Sara acting out her projected indifference with two desultory performances, a potential talent settling for seventy percent. Freshman Aidan circled around and around in his first 3200 meter, trying to figure out how he should feel and pace. He survived no worse for the experience of ballooning lap times. And I watched the boys 4x200 relay, without one of their key members, still finish 2nd and lay down a marker for future improvements. Parents and spectators lined the balcony railing above, either peering down intently or chatting up neighbors. And on the bus back to the high school later, the athletes were chattering too, the airwaves full of plans and hopes for the holiday break that had just begun.

***

Late in December, Coach P. was not happy. We talked after practice, and he complained that his workout was crappy. The athletes ran their sprint intervals with lackluster efforts--all of them. For a guy who can usually find something positive in a day's coaching, nothing about our early-morning vacation practice pleased him. So, we deconstructed his workout a bit, and I allowed that when I come off a break or a weekend, as we just had, I usually conduct the strength types of training. Experience has demonstrated that it's impractical to expect precision from the athletes on those days. "So maybe I should have run the longer intervals?" he wondered. "Yeah, probably," I told him.

Mine, on the other hand, generally pleased me. I should have been in a sour mood because Matt was bothered by a minor injury and could not handle much of our Monte Vista steep hill ascents. One other runner was still out with knee problems and another absent due to an appointment. Cindy was away on a family vacation, while Terri and Dave were no-shows. Tom, earlier, had notified me he would be missing our early morning practice due to "a family issue." Add to that Pam, who was practicing but taking it easier due to a slight injury. Her favorite training buddy, Sara, now had a ready-made excuse to moderate her own efforts. We call those slowdown decisions "sympathy paces." So, in that clear, calm twenty-two degree morning on Monte Vista, I had enough reasons to be dissatisfied.

Instead, they accomplished a lot of hard work. Matt reached his safe limit after a few intervals, and we decided he'd finish with twenty minutes at general conditioning pace around the top loop floating above the neighborhoods below. "Matt," I told him half-way into his time, "You are the first in the history of Wildcats Indoor Track to run a GC atop Monte Vista." Pleased, he smiled and plugged on. Everyone ultimately ran slightly slower paces than during an earlier version of the workout, but it was, after all, the first day back after four away on our mini-break for the athletes—and a cold morning to boot.

As we finished, an old retiree came out from his nearby house. He was walking his lawn, inspecting, checking on things. When he spied me, I waved and complimented him on the length of his immense flag-pole. The thing soared above his yard shrubs, challenging the border trees. The retiree wandered into the street and, as the runners finished and trudged down the hill to record times and jog back to the high school, we chatted. He told me all about that flagpole, why it was so damn tall.

Jackson

The arctic express was right on schedule. This day had broken open with a brittle sunshine that sparked the white fields aside Howlett Hill Road. I was running a little late for an early 8:00 a.m. team practice, and the dashboard thermometer read a frozen 12o. Meteorologists had already warned that we would not break the 20o mark, day or night, for eleven more days. We had slipped into the deep freeze.

I turned right onto Kasson Road and drove it down toward snowy drumlins and the Ontario lake plains that stretched beyond into an azure haze. Nearing a West Genesee Street shopping plaza, I saw a solitary runner plugging ahead on the road's right shoulder. He was carrying a small backpack that bounced with each stride, his breaths puffing out rhythmically white, like a steam locomotive. A brave soul, I first thought, but then quickly realized that the short, stocky frame and stilted stride looked all too familiar.

It's a funny thing. There are runners whose faces have long passed beyond my powers of recollection, but if I see them from a distance, out on a run, I'll say, *oh, there's Leslie* or *that's gotta be Ryan*, all of my former team members with strides irrefutable for identification, a runner's form of finger-printing. There was certainly no mistaking Jackson's bobbing and tilted build, as though always readying to duck a punch. He was huffing toward to the high school to make practice on time—and it was going to be close. I turned into the post office lot, dropped my letters into an outside mailbox and circled back onto Kasson. By then, Jackson had veered into the shopping plaza and was angling his way through the early cars parked in front of Walmart. Anything, he was surely calculating, to shorten the frigid commute.

Instead of continuing to West Genesee Street, I pulled around into the Walmart lot, maneuvered my way into the next parking lane beyond Jackson and stopped. He wove between two vehicles, then came up short as he recognized my car. His round face glowed red from the cold. With a hand wave, I motioned him around to the passenger side, then powered down the window. He stood there, starring and breathing heavily.

"Where you coming from?" I asked.

"My grandmother's," he said simply, as though that was all I needed to know.

"So, where's that?"

Jackson's reply was confusing, but I calculated about a mile and a half back up and off Kasson. And still at least a half mile to go.

I leaned over and popped the passenger side door open. He just stood there patiently, ruddy-faced and still breathing hard, as though I didn't mean anything by the gesture.

"Jackson," I finally told him, "get in."

January

We stood on our low window ledge during warm-ups, and I grumbled about all the "Family Vacation" absences during the holiday break. Coach P. simply nodded and recalled what an old principal of his had once told staff: "You can't teach an empty desk." Every year, I purposely built a 4-5 day break for the athletes into the holiday vacation. They had their training assignments, of course, but every year, some athletes and their parents ignored the plan, taking their days off when they damn well felt like it. Theirs was a distinct minority, to be sure, but always just enough of them caused mental aggravation. You can't, after all, coach an MIA athlete any better than you can teach an empty desk.

The runners filed by--some faster than others—on their 12 minute Monday morning hallway warm-up. It was a crisp 22° beyond the plate glass, but with only a light breeze and nothing falling. That meant the middle-distance runners were heading out to The Rise, our sloping 220 meter neighborhood road incline perfect for faster intervals and strength development. Our next meet lay only five days away, and two athletes who had returned from extended ten-day vacation sojourns weren't even among those circling our "L" hallway. Based on their complaints after attendance, I'd sent both right to the trainer, who diagnosed them too injured to train. That was a head-scratcher. Neither had been injured before their vacation departure, so the question was how they managed to mess themselves up laying on beaches. Neither could provide a suitable answer, but their 81% and 54% practice attendance averages told me I might just want to put coaching efforts elsewhere. My former colleague, Coach Delsole, had once told his athletes on another team, *Don't worry if I'm yelling. I'm just trying to make you a better athlete. When I stop yelling, then you can worry. It means I've given up.* I understood the sentiment.

Jackie came striding by, passing the slower flow of runners. When she circled back, I stopped her. "Jackie," I said down her from my slightly elevated perch on the low marble window ledge, "would you like to go to a state championship in the 4x400?" I didn't even give her enough time to be perplexed with that out-of-the-blue question. "I have not put you down as a possible member of our 4x400 because— to be honest—I did not know if your heart would be in it." Jackie starred back, wordless. So I kept going. "Would you think about it?" She agreed to that and headed back to her warm-up buddies.

Extending the vision of runners, getting kids to 'think big,' or at least bigger, is part of the job. For some athletes, it's asking a lot; they have developed their habitual comfort zones. But because it is always wrong to assume a runner's intentions, you keep asking those kind of questions. As often as not, those think-big suggestions are simply long casts into the wide waters of possibilities, hoping for a bite.

Later, after I'd returned from our middle-distance workout on The Rise and was watching my distance squad click off 4x200 meters at race pace on our indoor hallway oval, I saw Jackie again. Her sprinters group was conducting an indoor pyramid workout, and Jackie had just powered over the line after a 400 meter interval. As she bent for a breath, I asked, "Would you want to race on that 4x400?"

Jackie could have delivered the *I don't know* expression or simply made something up. But she was candid and told me she didn't seem to be able to muster "the push" for that distance. I thought about that while my distance group rested and the sprinters completed their final 400 meter interval. Jackie came through the first 200m lap trailing one of the boys' runners by about 10 meters. "Do it, Jackie!"

I shouted as she powered down the front straight. When she came around for the finish, she had caught and passed that boy. I offered my congratulations. "You know," I said to her, "you are able to 'flick the switch' and just go." She nodded tiredly. She even grinned a little.

School came back in session, and that first January afternoon I planned to take the middle-distance squad to our upstairs high school hallways for practice. Three features of that building area work well for the runners. The first attraction is a one hundred-twenty-meter long hallway, straight as an arrow, perfect for shorter forms of speed play and just wide enough to accept pairs of athletes coming and going. My runners have also developed an acquired taste for the quirky 354-meter circular passage that links all the different short halls up there, something we affectionately call The Grand Prix. During runs through that maze, I stand at the one place where I can sight up and down the long hall while still seeing some of the back halls through a linking passage. We counted the corners once—nine, and not all in the same direction--hence the name. But what I really like about that upstairs realm is the quiet. It's mostly empty in the afternoons, so nobody bothers us. Out of sight, out of mind. Our congenial janitorial staff has taken to positioning their cleaning carts so as not to totally block the halls. The occasional late-leaving teacher will stand off to the side as runners whoosh by, smiling or maybe even laughing and waving to a student we share. Most days, the middle-distance runners prefer to be outside, but there are those particular afternoons when the weather is just too abominable or when we need solitary precision in a climate-controlled setting. That's when we head upstairs to our quiet haven.

Up there, I always remember the old days when our previous superintendent banned us from using any hallways in the entire district. It was the same superintendent who had orchestrated the cutting of Indoor Track years earlier during an austerity year. And it was the same administrator who was unable, a half decade later--to block Indoor Track's eventual reinstatement by the Board of Education because we had so few winter sports options for girls. So that hallway ban could just have been out of spite. He eventually left for another state and an opportunity to increase his retirement pension. We went back to our secluded upstairs hallways. Sometimes I tell my runners that story--as a reminder.

Before practice, when I announced the plan to head up, several of the distance athletes immediately smiled and offered their indoor forecast: threshold run on the Grand Prix. And when I said "it's a combi day," Matt chirped: "and 20-10-30-5." There would be speed work tacked on to their precision running.

Beneath the thick, translucent glass block windows of a connector hallway, I delivered some rah-rah about why everyone needed to nail their target threshold paces, Outside, the temperature was falling fast, with rising winds and snow, but that would matter for nothing in our quiet, angled hallways. I set them off in small groups and walked up the long hallway to my typical position to call out the accumulating time. Their job was to count their laps and, of course, keep pace during the twenty minutes around their nine corners.

It was just bad luck that Tammi was still sick and out of school. She and Pam would have paired nicely to match paces and support each other. Cindy was game, so she and Pam started together. Threshold runs, though, are not interval workouts, where runners get to re-group after efforts of shorter distances. In these runs, any slight difference in aerobic capabilities or mindset will soon result in gaps between runners. The gaps grow and, at some point, groups of unequal aerobic abilities or willpower fragment. With this training, you don't, of course, want runners to race in order to keep up, so except on teams blessed by a core of like abilities, gaps are predictable.

Matt, our outlier, expected to run alone, but after him followed a chase pack of three--Steve, Aidan and Justin--that held together most of the twenty minutes. Behind them trailed Pam and Cindy, with Sara a little further off at a slightly slower pace. Another disjointed group of guys followed, and behind them, Terri and Nancy plied the halls at wary speeds.

For the first five minutes, everyone strode smartly in their groups down the long hall past me before veering left and disappearing into the back hallways. I shouted the minutes in halves: "Eight minutes gone!" or "Coming on ten!" They motored and kept track of their .22 mile Grand Prix laps. Around and around. Afternoon light wanned through the glass block windows as I watched passing expressions and strides, looking for those tell-tale posture signs beyond the obvious changing gaps between runners. Then Pam appeared at the end of the long hall alone. Cindy had dropped back to run with Sara. As she passed, Pam mumbled something I didn't understand, but I knew it meant she had locked into a pace she refused to relinquish, one which Cindy chose not to sustain. "Fine," I answered, and instructed her to keep the boys chase pack, about twenty meters ahead, as close as possible. Cindy came around with Sara, while the others held their groups and positions. Twelve minutes on the clock; eight remaining. Around and around. They ran through their sweet spots of balanced efforts and chosen expectations, into the harder finishing minutes. I called out the minutes and then the remaining time. Runners churned by. When I whistled their twenty minutes up, runners in the long hall pulled up, hands on hips. Other groups slowly reappeared from the hidden hallways. After a short break and water, everyone massed at one end of the long hall, ready to switch to the other side of the endurance/speed spectrum.

Coach Jack Reed, of nearby Skaneateles High School, had devised the workout. Coach Delsole, once his assistant, then mine, brought the workout with him. Coach Reed had used an even longer hallway in his high school, but ours was long enough. The 20-10-30-

5 moniker referred to the recovery seconds allowed between sprints up and down the hall. Five sprints, four too-brief rests. That was a set. What my runners thought ingenious was the shortest five-second rest—basically a deep breath, a turn, and go—had been placed prior to the last and hardest sprint. Ingenious in a diabolical way.

Our runners would always complete two sets, sometimes three, depending. Unlike the threshold run, where we could convert distance and laps into comparable per/mile paces, I never logged any times on their 20-10-30-5 sets. I just told tell to start and stop their own watches to see if they could make each set go faster. Typically, that happened with the veteran runners, and so it was always inspiring to watch tired athletes at the end of a workout amping up their efforts and speed, down that narrow, half-lit, quiet high school hallway, the only sounds their heavy breathing and the whoosh of feet through the corridor. For most, finishing faster was more than a habit. It was a matter of pride.

They powered up and down the hallway, hunched between efforts, with little small-talk. Sometimes, as the recovery seconds ticked off, someone would utter "let's go" to the others with a slight hand wave. Sometimes, the group would simply step to the start together and communally fire off. The veteran coaches and physiologists can explain at length the benefits of using this type of speed at the end of the day to improve muscle recruitment when tired. For my runners, it was also mimicking the demands of any long race where you try to hold pace with mounting fatigue. For a final time, they zoomed to my end of the hall—the 5 second end—heaved a breath as they turned and launched out on their last sprint. At the far end, their hard work finished, they bent over and sucked oxygen.

Once they finished their cool-down laps and stretches, the runners disappeared down the stairwell with their easy conversations and benign banter. I gathered up the med kit and my clipboard. Quiet settled back into the empty upper hallways. Outside, the wind whistled its lonesome tune.

***

Brimming with Google Maps confidence, I directed the bus driver away from his preferred route and along residentials streets to a supposedly faster back entrance to the Utica College Athletic Center bubble. Glenn, the driver, had tilted his head slightly while taking my altered instructions and said, "I just hope there's no locked gate." We were running a little late; this shortcut was going to save the early-event athletes some valuable warm-up time. And besides, Google Maps and I had guided him through all the important turns of our country approach once off the Thruway at Westmoreland. What could he know that me and Google Maps didn't?

Enough, as it turned out. We maneuvered down to the final street, sighting the huge white bubble of the athletic center rising in the background above the neighborhood. Then, cresting a slight rise, we slowly approached the chained road gate with a huge red STOP sign anchored in its middle. Glenn didn't say anything as he managed to turn the bus around, find a way back to Burrstone Road and follow other buses through the usual entrance. He could have said some things, but he didn't.

This meet was a track and field version of Friday Night Lights. Our arcane central New York sport had come a long way. The dark days of Section III Indoor Track & Field began in 2017 when Syracuse University decided to no longer offer its Manley Field House indoor track for high school meets. Indoor football practice space was what they wanted in that facility, so someone—us--had to go. Without a central meet site, our sport faced an imminent threat to its existence—and there were even voices suggesting just that, to do away with Section III Indoor Track. Rather than throw in the towel, a small number of obstinate old-timers patched together several seasons that required long bus rides to other rented indoor tracks at colleges in the area. We survived just long enough. Even as my own parents beat back an attempt by our former school officials to cut the sport, the forward thinkers at Onondaga Community College were completing their Sports and Recreation Center, a place containing the indoor track facility that our Section III West schools would soon call home. Our area of the section, Section III West, was divided into six groups, each containing 6-7 schools, and the groups competed against each other in rotation during Saturday morning and afternoon invitational sessions at the college.

And then, the sport that some critics claimed was unsustainable and on its last legs began growing. It grew so rapidly that, within a few years athletes, coaches and officials had trouble fitting everyone in. With a 200 meter 6-lane track, long and triple jump pit, pole vault and high jump areas, shot put and weight-throw arcs, and the remaining infield taken up with team spots--there was no unused space on the arena floor. Meanwhile, the twenty-plus schools in Section III East that had still been using one of our former dark-years college facilities, moved into Utica College's new Athletic Center. Their home domain was now a spacious realm of eight track lanes, multiple jump pits and an entire indoor lacrosse/football field at the back end to be used as team sites during meets. To alleviate our own OCC crunch, for each meet one of the Section III West groups would bus down the Thruway to compete instead in the East's Friday night competitions. This night it was our turn.

Glenn edged the bus around the back of the arena, and we queued before the large airlock entrance for athletes and heavy equipment. A pair of eyes peered out through a plastic portal and the outside garage-like door creaked open. Once crammed into the passageway with several other school teams, the outer door closed and the inside door raised to the bustling and brightly lit interior of the dome. We'd arrived no worse for my navigating.

The team found an open spot on the practice field and settled in. JV Sprint Medley Relay athletes and our entries in the 3200 and 3000 boys/girls first varsity events all jogged away on warmups while I walked to the scorers' table for the coaches' meeting. The evening was underway.

Matt and teammate Aidan were our first varsity racers to toe the start-line in the 3200 meter race. As a first-season indoor guy, Aidan was still learning the competitive track distances. He had arrived as a neophyte cross-country member in August with a modest two hundred eighty miles of summer training under his belt. Then he pushed himself too relentlessly and lost the second half of that season to injury. Indoor was a second chance, an opportunity to manage a competitive season correctly—and to have an impact on the team. Aidan had already completed almost a complete survey of the middle-distances, racing the 4x800, 1600, and 3200 meter events. Now, we began the process of identifying his strongest race distance with his second shot at the long one.

Not surprisingly, Matt pushed out quickly. With two previous attempts at that distance, he was adjusted to its demands and hoped to break the ten-minute mark for the first time. He had raced the distance only the week before but successfully lobbied to violate our typical protocol of alternating races distances. I should have choreographed his sequence better, and I should have known he had a specific competitor in mind. That Adirondack racer he would face only twice in the season, was savvy. Knowing his competition, he lurked patiently behind Matt, allowing him the mental pressure of holding the lead. They were, at that moment, the early show under the lights. Halfway through the sixteen laps, sensing a stagnating pace, his rival surged past Matt, built a workable lead and eventually won.

His winning time, however, was slower than Matt's two previous efforts. Matt just shook his head, while I mentally kicked myself. Aidan, meanwhile, improved by five seconds and raced the second fastest freshman time of the meet. His race tactics, though, left him disappointed with his performance. He expected better but got a pat on the back for the effort.

As the meet moved along, Coach P. and I bustled around, making sure athletes clerked in, recording laps times for the distance runners and relays, checking the field events athletes. I had looked forward to Sandy's 600 meter race, and the first heats of that event were already queuing on the infield. The distance was a calculated race experiment for Sandy, a sprint-type athlete with a big heart and steely determination. Sandy had always displayed solid 200 to 400 meter speed but not top sectional capabilities at those distances. The year before, I had proposed to her that we try extending her race range to include the 600 meter. Sandy gave it thought and agreed. I had no concern about her commitment to the project. Half-measures were not Sandy's style. In her sophomore year, she had given up Marching Band to run cross-country for added strength and to teach some of those intermediate muscle types to operate more aerobically. Success in the 600 had come slowly, but Sandy was persistent and demanding. As she waited on the infield for her fast heat, I remembered an indoor race of hers the previous year, also in the Utica College dome. That night, following her 300 meter effort, I had located her on the infield, staring at the floor as though deep in thought. I held up my hand to offer a high-five as I approached because she had, after all, just run her seasonal best time in that event. But she shook her head no and waved me off. "That was awful!" she blurted. "I can do much better!" I had lowered my hand, given her a pat on the shoulder and walked away.

This night, she stepped up to the start line with several of the top sectional runners at that distance. Two of them would eventually qualify for the state championship. With the gun, Sandy charged out and tucked in behind the top seed, a racer from Central Valley. Her sprinter's race imperative, as always, was to compress the lap times as much as possible. A shrinking range between fastest and slowest laps would simply indicate she had effectively controlled her anerobic speed inclinations and maximized the use of that hard-won aerobic ability. Previously, I had watched her blow up in several races, going out too fast, exuberant with her fast-twitch muscle energy, then hitting the proverbial wall as she depleted that source of speed too quickly and lurched the final lap home on wooden legs. Pace control was primary. Sandy's innate desire needed to be tempered by discipline, and we were never exactly sure how far we could take the experiment.

The racers barreled into lap two, with Sandy still secure in the second spot, charging ahead of another talented racer from Central Square who had already beaten her once in December. That middle lap, for Sandy, was like the jet pilot checking all the gauges before an airport approach. Body mechanics, race position, mental relaxation with the established speed—this was the critical lap where, if the checks were positive, an excellent race was possible with a strong closing lap. Sandy came through under a second slower than her first lap—a positive indicator of controlled pacing. And she was in the mix. That competitive distance, like an 800 meter contested correctly, is never about finishing faster. It's about controlling the inevitable slowing with increased effort. The athlete who slows the least runs the most effective race and, if talented, sometimes wins. I held my breath during Sandy's third lap because I knew the physiological tightrope she walked. I knew what could happen. But Sandy was simply into the race, emersed by that magic moment when, unburdened by notions of greatness, greatness sometimes arrives. She bore down with her big heart, controlled her mechanics and held off the Central Square racer to place second with a personal record and her smallest

[57]

lap range ever. Few in the arena would notice, but with smart tactics, discipline and guts, it was the closest yet she had come to a perfect race.

There were other small, private victories by team athletes that evening. And there were disappointments. The meet was, in that way, typical. But when Dan and Jake and Pat and Easais squared off against a Proctor 4x200 meter relay that held one of the state's current top times--and placed a close second with a new school record--Coach P. and I knew those four seniors had suddenly announced an arrival. They were in the mix.

***

The sprinters shuffled down from their upstairs hallway short intervals practice as mid-January weather blustered outside. They had only to complete a final two lap all-out effort on our 200 meter lower hall oval. My distance group had filled the oval for most of the afternoon, running an 'uncertainty interval' workout where they never knew the length of their next interval until lined up. Their last effort, though, could usually be guessed: something speedy to "finish fast." So no one had been surprised when I announced their 400m. As they speed around, I ushered the sprinters into the open space of our start area. They watched the distance crew muscle the tight corners and pull up, exhausted, bending over with hands on knees. Now it was their turn.

Coach P. lined them up for their unenviable 400-meter task. As I complimented my distance members on a good day's work, Coach P. launched the sprinters. They circled once, then bore down into their second and final lap. We stopped to cheer them down the long front hall, then waited for them to circle around. Most powered through their final turn and crossed the finish where they slumped, fatigued but pleased with their efforts--and even more pleased to be done. I glanced over the bent bodies and then down the short side hall. There came Lily around the last corner, walking her final meters. She seemed unconcerned about being caught strolling. And right behind her, smiling, was Jenna playfully pushing Lily, as though providing a neighborly assist. Seeing me, they increased their speed to a shameless shuffle. I was amazed. I simply watched.

Someone once created a four-box rubric for coaches, one that conceptualizes the basic 'types' of athletes that coaches are likely to encounter in their careers. The rubric reminds us of the wide range of athletes who inevitably arrive in no-cut sports like track or cross-country. Movement along the horizontal axis of that rubric, left to right, indicates increasing skills and talent. Movement up the vertical axis, bottom to top, indicates increasing motivation. The 'types' of athletes are thus mixtures of talent and motivation.

The upper right Box 1 contains those athletes of high skills and high motivation. Those are the dream athletes who arrive infrequently for most coaches, and they are the ones we enjoy recalling in subsequent years. Directly below those dream athletes, in the lower right Box 2, are the team members of less skill but high motivation. Those athletes are the reasons most of us continue coaching season after season, year after year. They enjoy the sport and its challenges. They make valuable contributions, and many are inspirational.

If coaching was limited to athletes in those two boxes, everyone would sleep soundly. But there are two other boxes. In the above left-hand Box 3 sit those athletes of superior talent but low motivation. They are the cause of many coaching regrets. They make us second guess; they leave us wondering *what if?* You learn to live with these kinds of athletes, though. You learn how to lose some of them, too, because sometimes the only choice, for their sake and the team, is to let go. Coach Oscar Jensen, a dean of local and state coaches, once told me my favorite Box 3 story. "So, I was having a really hard time once with a thrower," he said, "A talented kid, but he just wouldn't make it to all the practices. Finally, the kid shows up one day after missing another workout, so I pulled him aside. I got another excuse, so I said to him, 'Listen, why don't you just take two weeks off—then quit.'" Of course, we all go on coaching missions, attempting to support or sway faltering or disinterested athletes, trying repeatedly to turn on the light. And more often than not, those missions fail, and names get added to the what-might-have-been list. Just enough of them, though, succeed to ensure future missions.

The last, Box 4, in the lower left, is the coach's head-scratcher list. These are the team members of low skills and low motivation, young adults who often appear purposeless or intent on majoring only in minor things. They are typically good kids, but for whatever reasons, the sport you are attempting to introduce isn't worth their full effort or their daily time. Coach Delsole and I once watched such a team member slog through another workout at the back of the pack with another half-effort, all the while sporting a pained expression. We had already run through the gamut of interventions—and nothing had worked. He simply shook his head. "Really," he said, "I don't know why he keeps showing up." Sometimes, of course, they keep showing up because all those purposeless efforts serve the purpose of beating the alternative places to be. And that's a sad, low bar.

Use of the four-box matrix is handy but flawed. Its assumption of mean-averages in each box(e.g. high skills/low motivation always results in minimal success) assumes the permanence of conditions. But low motivation can improve. The high skills of an athlete can deteriorate due to chronic injuries or even maturation. For adolescents, what the model and its predictive boxes requires is time and its opportunity for change—second chances, third chances, fourth. Coaches who do not have that element of time (i.e. sports with tryouts and cuts) or coaches inclined to believe athletes are not capable of change—those coaches will judge team members on present conditions instead of potential futures.

I starred at Lilly, who had attended one of our six holiday practices, seven of our last sixteen, and then at Jenna, her congenial but unmotivated side-kick I had once driven home from a late meet because her mother simply did not show or answer her phone. Jenna, Lilly and I—we'd also had our talks to no effect. They were on their third chance--or was it fourth? That might have been the moment to launch into a lecture in front of their teammates, if only to provide an object lesson. But there was no point. The worst team infraction is not to hate running. A fair number of our neophytes—and even a few of our veterans over time—decide they hate running. And you can sympathize because there is a lot of pain involved. No, the worst infraction is a refusal to take it seriously. That is a direct affront to those who do, and who wants a teammate around day after day who lacks any seriousness about the endeavor to which you've devoted heart and soul? Indifferent athletes make the worst teammates, and after multiple attempts to create investment, a coach is well advised to either remove that athlete from the team or find a way to insulate the others.

I glanced at those other runners recovering from the intervals and sprints of the day. Some were wearily recording times; others were patting teammates on the back or offering fist-bumps. They all seemed oblivious to those two among them, still fresh from doing nothing. No one was discourteous, no one disdainful nor dismissive— just oblivious. They had already protected themselves. So I turned to them instead.

January 2018

The alarm went off at 4:56 a.m. I dressed in the dark, tip-toed down the steps and eased out the side door into the cold morning. Plow trucks plied the shadowy roads on my drive to the high school. The temperature hovered around 10°, a now empty sky making way for falling temperatures. I pulled left off West Genesee Street into the school's upper circle and veered left again down to the lower lot, vacant except for a district utility truck by the small maintenance room. I parked, and, with the engine running for heat, I waited. Without a high school security card, I had to meet--and walk in with--the morning custodian when he opened up at 5:30 a.m.

In a few minutes, car headlights poked their way off the street and down to the lower lot. I'd already locked my car and scuttled to the entrance, feeling the air's bite. A hunched figure straightened out of his car and shuffled to the door where I waited.

"Morning Jimbo," I said.

"Uhmmmm...," he mumbled as he opened the door and went into janitor's room to turn off the school's alarm system. "Jimbo" was loved by the students; he just wasn't what you'd consider a morning person.

"Have a good one Jimbo," I told him as I passed on my way to the stairs.

"Uhmmmm...," Jimbo said.

The building sat in a dimly lit silence, and it was a short walk up to the main floor, along and around Cafeteria II, then past the other cafeteria to the Weight Room. I wedged the door open with an old cast iron plate and turned on the lights. The room was chilly; custodians had obviously dialed down the thermostat for that part of the building to cut energy costs. I left on a fleece top to start my twenty-five minutes of stationary biking before the athletes arrived.

Around six a.m., the first kids stomped in. Security procedures dictated that I should meet each of them at the pool entrance, but that would have meant unsupervised athletes in one part of the building while I was waiting for others in another. So I had them trudge around the back of the building to the Weight Room's outside doors where they could either bang twice for entrance, or, if lucky, find one of the doors wedged off its lock just enough for them to finger it open. Then they'd tromp in with school and athletic backpacks burdening their shoulders, give me a wave if I was still biking, stamp the snow off boots and sign in before starting their exercise routines.

We called ourselves "The Risers," and for the second year a resolute group of team members had Tuesday/Thursday workouts to start their school days in the wee hours. We also had some parents to thank for that.

The day's group included Matt, Natalie, Joe, Tony, Katie, Abby, Chris, Taylor, Jack, Aubrey and Emily. They set about with the Tuesday routine Coach Mosatti, our strength guru, had specifically designed for distance runners. Coach M's Thursday's routine addressed slightly different muscle groups. All the kids had the exercises down, and if someone forgot, others were there with reminders. I finished my cycling and circulated among the athletes before starting some strength work myself. Bob Deegan, a science teacher and Varsity lacrosse assistant, had arrived and begun his 'cardio day,' but not before wandering over with his patented greeting: "Hey Jim, gotta joke for ya." "Deegs" was a weight room fixture, a workout maven, and probably the most highly qualified assistant lacrosse coach in state history, the defensive specialist on a legendary program with a legendary head coach. Deegs had turned down head coaching offers from other schools and could have worked on the collegiate level if he chose. He was that good. As he huffed on his stationary bike, plugged into headphones, a few others wandered in—baseball and lacrosse players prepping for the spring season, and another teacher staying in shape. Someone had cranked the radio up a few notches, and the music blended with the clang of barbell weights, athletes groaning out the last seconds of core positions and the thwap of our heavy ropes being rhythmically snaked up and down. The place hummed in contrast to the silent halls that waited patiently for their morning rush hour.

And just as gradually as the room had taken life, athletes finished, shouldered packs and left, sneaking out the hubbub with them. Deegs had a science lesson to arrange, so he finished early and waved goodbye. I straightened up workout sheets, replaced some of the weights left scattered, turned off the music and the lights, and closed the door behind me. On the walk out, I passed the early arriving teachers and food service folks setting up for the day. Jimbo was still making his morning rounds, nowhere to be seen. The morning cold was even more brittle as I slowly motored home. Turning left and driving down Onondaga Boulevard, the sun had just come peeking through the city silhouettes in the distance, lighting the undersides of a few refugee clouds. Traffic had picked up. People were rushing toward their days.

***

The work so far, and the seasonal progressions, indicated the runners were ready go at it faster. Our Monday interval workout had been solid, followed by Tuesday recovery running in the neighborhood. For this midweek practice, they were inside for the last hard work out before Saturday's meet. I introduced a new session: Flying 50's. The typical presentation of this speed-interval workout consists of 2x1600 meters with 50-meter sprint zones interspersed with 50 meters of 'float' for recovery while maintaining some speed. I broke it down into 4x800 because the sprint zones fit nicely into our long hallway segments of The Oval, with the short halls and turns used for the 'float' meters. "Just record totals for each 800," I told them to keep things simple. That way they could compare times with future efforts. Improvements would come with either better sprint speed or ability to 'float' more quickly. Either improvement would demonstrate they were becoming faster racers.

The school was humming with activity—basketball in the upper gym, wrestlers in their downstairs padded room, the swimmers in the pool and volleyball in the smaller lower gym. Coach Corley had the weight room bustling with off-season football players, so I kept an eye out for any of his athletes wandering into the hall where my runners pushed their zones. Sandy and Rob had been plucked from their sprint groups to join us. This workout would hone their sprint endurance.

The popular jargon celebrates the "safe haven" that running provides its practitioners. "Best part of your day," I had often found

[65]

myself jesting to school-weary athletes. The truth is that most can't simply leave their days behind at dismissal. Enthusiasm for our work is always the expectation, but not all of a bad school day can be discarded or ignored. A significant challenge of some training days is not the work itself, but the mind that must be rallied to the cause. Decisions on effort are sometimes the product of influences beyond the runners' control, though sometimes runners do simply make choices.

It didn't take long to judge who was going to dig into the work and who, having run the calculations and made a decision, might hold back mentally and physically. And so, where Justin had 'fallen off the wagon' during a disappointing Monday effort, this afternoon he was pushing for all he was worth, as though determined to atone. Cindy, however, seemed to decide she simply did not have 'it' this day. Down and around the afternoon hallways, she watched Pam, Tammi and Sandy slowly pull away in the first set, and then she settled back in with Sara. Those two ran not far off the front group, but just far enough. The expression of desire in this type of work is revealed in distances.

Matt, after only a few laps, was solo as usual, but the runner usually closest in pursuit, Aidan, was now joined by Jack, Steve, and our sprinter Rob. So there was Jack, in the thick of the chase group again instead of languishing further back. More than once, he had left me scratching my head—but in a good way. His potential was apparent. In workouts, he typically timed second or third of the boys. In meets, however, he seldom stood out, creating quiet or desultory performances, just the way he often appeared in person. The job was to infuse that innate talent with competitive desire. It had been tough task.

They gave their best for the day, which for most was all that was expected. Around and around they circled, leaning into the sprint zones, gliding out of them. The afternoon light paled through the hallway windows. When they finally pulled up, group by group, some bent over gasping while others walked in crooked circles, hands on hips, breathing deeply. Not all had mastered the work, but all had at least managed it. Justin's Monday blues had disappeared. Lagging in that tough third set, he had borne down in the last, which became his fastest. After I instructed the groups on their cool-down run, he walked over with a question. "Coach, is there a chance I can make the league championship squad?" I explained that Coach P. and I were still deciding on the two allowed individual entries in each event, entries typically decided by the cold calculus of the stopwatch.

But that was mostly a ruse. Mentally, I had already penciled him in.

***

The schools were racing each other in our final invitational before the championships, and all of us were racing the snow. A big storm was projected to envelop central New York late afternoon and into the evening. Over 50% of the schools entered in the afternoon session of the Grieve Memorial had preemptively cancelled. The white deluge wouldn't stop, forecasters announced, until Sunday afternoon, twelve to twenty-four inches later. Then bitter cold would drop like a steel curtain, and Monday would be zero and wind-whipped. Monday, though, was the MLK holiday, so the schools would have time to dig out and keep the bus batteries functional.

Our morning session was proceeding, but the start had been pushed up an hour, so the athletes were a little bleary-eyed for our team bus departures. I cut the leave time as close as possible to leave warm-up time for the 8:00 a.m. meet start, but we still almost left three girls behind, all who boarded just before the door closed with gazes averted from their irritated coach and not so much as a "Sorry." The miracle occurred on the other bus, where all the boys were in their seats and ready to pull out on time.

A light snow, as though unintentional, fell as we stepped from our buses at the OCC arena. Inside, the floor was already busy with athletes, coaches, and staff. My former coaching partner, Coach Delsole, greeted us as we set up a team area. Now retired, he was assisting with clerking athletes due to the absence of officials. This was the fourth invitational those sectional officials had been on strike over a dispute about the method of work payments. Most coaches

[68]

had heard rumors of their reasons for striking, but nothing from the officials themselves. The coaching reactions had been varied.

For the athletes, though, the meets had gone on as normal. A few throwers had grumbled that their distances were incorrectly marked, and one indignant team member at the previous week's meet showed me a video of a competitor running out of lane during a relay exchange, a transgression that went unnoticed by the volunteer official. Mostly, however, the season had progressed properly--and no one had been denied an event or a meet due to the strike. Nothing but upstate weather had been able to accomplish that.

The JV SMR athletes shook off sleep and lined up, waiting for the gun and the mayhem that only their mass event can produce. Coaches leaned on the track-side crowd rails with stopwatches because those non-varsity events were their responsibility to time. We had only one boy's squad but two and a half girls relays, that half due to team members who emailed us the night before with their particular illnesses. The boys squads charged off the line, with relay baton exchanges a loosely controlled confusion of bumping bodies and twirling arms. I glanced up to the spectator balcony where parents queued against the rail to watch their youngster churn out a brief competitive moment--and I wondered what they thought. Were they pleased and proud for their kid's opportunity to train and compete? Or blasé to the offering? Could they imagine beyond the brief seconds here on the track to the long afternoons of sweaty effort in narrow halls or snow-bordered roads where the real value lay for their kids? It was impossible to know, but worth wondering.

Coach P. had disappeared to his assignment of helping record attempts at the Pole Vault event, but he shortly returned. "They didn't need me," he reported with some satisfaction. Which was fine by me; I certainly needed him to help with event lap splits. And he was now free to monitor his sprinters and field event athletes.

The rhythms of the meet took over even as we raced the

approaching storm. Three of our runners brought up the rear of the 3200 meter event, two of them plugging through difficult days, proving they were no 'morning larks' when it came to circadian rhythms. But Justin circled his sixteen laps with intent, building on a possibility. And in those third quarter laps, when runners often slow, Justin pushed faster. Others passed him, but he held on by working harder. The arms extended too much, even as his face remained expressionless and focused. In the final two laps, he pushed even harder.

***

When I returned home from a late January practice, there was an email for me. I read it while 15° winds swirled outside. Keri had written it only the hour before at home, while her teammates were all still hard at work in the high school hallways. She wanted me to understand her latest string of absences, but I already knew the reasons she'd been out of school for several weeks. *Hi coach,* she wrote. *I know I've been a little MIA lately. I've been struggling with some personal things that have unfortunately taken precedence to track and my schoolwork. Hopefully, I can get my act together for outdoor and make it a good one. I wanted to thank you for being so understanding and accommodating. Not just now but all throughout my running career. You brought me into this sport and I can't thank you enough for that. I don't know what's going to happen next season, but running with this team has been the best thing that's ever happened to me. And that wouldn't have been possible without you pushing me, and believing in me. You and this team have been my support whenever I needed it, and that's something I'll never be able to repay.*

I showed the email to my wife, who knew all about Keri's trials and tribulations. We both understood there was no rubric box to explain the troubles that girl was living. "That's nice," she said when she finished.

***

7:33a.m. Those students unfortunate enough to suffer early morning high school Regents exams are already sitting at desks in the main gym of the high school. Those others without exams--and thus the day off--are probably rolling over and mumbling goodbye to parents off to scrap snow from their car windows.

8:04a.m. I've checked the Leonetiming meet entries again for our Utica Challenge invitational this evening. Outside, it's a curious snow that just comes and goes. North up I-81, though, lake effect snow has choked the roads and deepened. It's still coming down hard between Syracuse and Watertown.

9:00a.m. A lot of schools in the eastern lee of Lake Ontario, the lake-effect districts, have surrendered and closed. Watertown, General Brown, Lowville, Pulaski—all done for the day. Weather radar paints a spindly snake of snow across the lake which fattens when it hits land, like someone pressing a white brush against dark canvas. Who gets what is a tricky call. Into or out of a meandering lake effect band is sometimes like stepping through a door. Our skies are mostly light clouds at the moment, though there's that second band snaking across the region, the one that's delivering the occasional moderate to heavy snow outside my study window. Weather Bug's hourly forecast claims "Partly Cloudy" most of the day. Really? Partly cloudy is simply the average of blizzard and sun. Our snow swath shoots west to east, meaning it extends down the Thruway over Rome and Oneida, all the way to Utica. If it gets comfortable there, if it decides to linger awhile, our Utica Challenge meet is in jeopardy.

9:36a.m. The northern list of closed schools grows longer, but here the snowfall has abated, so the danger for our district would have to

[72]

be an early dismissal if the snow bands twist. And early dismissal would mean no meet. We are not out of the woods yet.

9:50a.m. Sunlight is poking through thinning clouds.

11:49a.m. We have settled into clouds with random snowflakes drifting down. I e-mail 'final instructions' out to parents/athletes/coaches/AD. The winds are picking up as the temperature drops. The thermometer, says the hourly, will read 22° when we leave for Utica and 14° when we return. A late, cold ride home will end the day.

12:22p.m. The snow returns, wind-driven now instead of carelessly discarded by clouds. The temperature has dropped to 23°, beginning its long slide. Weather radar shows us back into the spindles of that lower CNY band. Things could change—storm to sun to storm again--in a matter of minutes. Sometimes that's how we live our winters.

12:35p.m. Sun's out. Shadows etch themselves in the backyards and driveways.

12:57p.m. A steady stream of colder crystalline snow has begun, but then the sun muscles through the light cloud cover again. Cold and blowy works for us. Cold and storm doesn't. Now, the 'window' for possible afternoon cancellation has shrunk to an hour. So far, most CNY schools have remained silent, and our invitational is still 'on.'

2:01p.m. Coach P. finishes exam proctoring and joins me in the hall by the pool entrance as athletes begin to arrive. We are a go. The unofficial headcount begins, and we know who to worry about.

2:24p.m. Our bus pulls up and the athletes board.

2:29p.m. Attendances complete, no one has run afoul our 'Miss-the-Team-Bus-Go-Home' rule. I sign the roster form for the driver and we're off.

2:41p.m. Stuck in an accident backup while still on I690 in Syracuse. The bus inches forward as minutes pass. Finally, we dart off a local exit and find the Carrier Circle Thruway entrance. Relieved to have built in some cushion time.

3:28p.m. The CNY uplands on the southern horizon seem stationary as the bus rocks and rolls along the Thruway. In the quickly passing snow-smoothed fields, the poked-up weed stubble all leans east.

[73]

3:55p.m. The bus drops us off at the double-door, air-lock athlete entrance, and we emerge into the bright lights of the field house bubble. With school cancellations, there's no shortage of team space on the back practice field. Those folks are all home watching snow pile up in their driveways. Our athletes are warming up for a long evening.

4:30-7:10p.m. Maybe it's the slow bus ride or the uncertainties of the day or maybe just the end of a long winter week, but the early events for team members don't go well. Justin and Steve in the 3200 meter, the girls or our 4x400, and the 55 meter sprinters—no one is notching a top time or personal record when that was the hope for a meet late in the regular season.

7:14p.m. Instantly, everything blows up. Jumped at her 600-meter start, Sandy traffics her way off the inside rail down the back-straight, but I can see the mind has already clicked into panic mode and the damage is done. Her internally calculated Hazard Score must be high, too high. Muscle memory and ingrained attitude forces the next two laps, but it's tears and disbelief after that. The time's not awful, but it's nowhere near what she expected of herself. "Sandy," I tell her with a pat on the shoulder, "I want you to take a short walk and then come back. I'll be right here."

7:39p.m. Following instructions and fighting the urge, Matt lays back, letting the 1600m front pack fight their fast battles while he reigns in false instincts. Discipline pays as laps click by with little fall-off in pace. He finds the right company, recognizes the win-able battles and, after a stinker lap 6, gathers and charges. A five second PR. An Open Qualifier standard. A good night.

8:35p.m. I find Riley near the long jump pit. She's beaming, so I ask. Entering her in the long jump event was almost an after-thought to her favored triple jump. But she's leaped a foot further than her previous best and only an inch shy of the sectional championship standard. Go figure.

9:05p.m. I find Tara's parents on the sideline, waiting for her final effort in the 4x200 that we'll get to eventually. We talk about her other sports specialty, soccer goalie, and I tell them again how athletically gifted their daughter is. "Push her," the father says, and I understand where a good chunk of her sports success comes from.

9:28p.m. An unknown runner almost leans into a false start of the 55 high hurdles, but the official quickly brings the field back up to a standing position for a reset. Good move. It reminds me of a 110 high hurdler years ago at the outdoor track state championship in Kingston. He was unable to catch his lean and was not rescued by any benevolent official. Disqualified, his head never lifted as he walked off the track. Hundreds of travel miles, months of time and preparation only to have his 12-13 second opportunity of a lifetime reduced to 0. Almost cruel.

10: 18p.m.: Our boys 4x200 has been among the section's best, but not this night. They finish out of the top 6 with a relay time that seems to be going backwards. Shaking heads and eye rolls. Something needs to change.

10:30p.m.: We have no one in the final event, the arcane 500 meter. I scan the parent sign-out list again and cross-check the meet sheet roster to ensure we have everyone back on our team bus. Not a good thing to leave someone behind. I know of a few coaches who have done just that. Embarrassment was the least result of their faux pas's.

10:39p.m.: Once through the airlock, our small, tired band boards the bus, and we roll out into the CNY darkness. "Call your parents that we're leaving the meet," I instruct them. "Tell them you will call again when we're off the thruway in Syracuse." Cell phones light up. Coach P. steers the driver out of the city.

11:19a.m.: Athletes doze in a silent bus as the cold country slips by. A half-moon drifts in and out of slivery clouds to the south.

11:44p.m.: A small miracle. One of the high school custodians is waiting for us as we curve into the lower parking lot, a parking lot thankfully full of waiting cars with engines running. Phil has graciously hung around, so I don't have to drive home with a vault pole stuck out my side window.

11:48p.m.: With gear stowed, Coach P. and I head to our cars, relieved by an empty lot and seeing no athletes waiting for wayward parents. "My ride's shorter," Coach had told me earlier, "I'll stay if necessary." But it looks like he's won this lottery. We both drive slowly around to the main entrance and, of course, there's one huddling on the sidewalk, waiting. Do the parents agree to take turns arriving late? Coach P parks nearby.

11:49p.m.: I pull up to our runner. "Where's your ride?" She looks at me, unfazed. "Oh, my mom took a nap while she was waiting. She's leaving now." How soon, I want to know. "Oh, she'll be here in ten or fifteen minutes." I look over at Coach in his car, settling in. God bless him.

12:13a.m.: The side door is unlocked and the kitchen light on. Marsha's upstairs in bed, and Harley won't even come down for a tail-wag greeting. I am not surprised.

Morgan

Before she graduated, Morgan confessed to me twice. The first was more of a pronouncement, uttered at a team meeting during one of her underclassman seasons. I had been talking about the athletes working harder, and amid the comments and complaints about my "unrealistic expectations," Morgan offered her own perspective on the matter. She declared I was "too obsessed with running," which was accompanied by agreeing, cautious nods of others and then a very long team discussion. Not much of their training changed, but the second confessional was more obliquely charitable when, nearing graduation, she jokingly disclosed that her mother used to think I was "trying to kill her."

By Morgan's senior year, my 'obsession' with running had somehow morphed to a less dangerous 'passion.' She qualified for the Cross-Country state championship that Fall as an individual runner, but on the Monday after sectionals was diagnosed by our trainer with a potential stress-fracture and referred for an MRI. At that point, I offered my condolences for such a cruel end to her final high school cross-country season, but Morgan cried and cajoled her mother into seeking a second opinion, finding a doctor willing to give her the week she needed "if she could stand the pain." With her parent's consent--and my doubts--she mostly rested, then gritted through her state championship, finishing 45th amid the cold Adirondack mountains.

Some runners come already tough, little shaping necessary. Most of those accept their toughness as a matter of stoic and practical fact, but a few oddballs find in it a manner of entertainment. After time off to heal, Morgan plunged into her senior indoor track season. It was a productive campaign, and at the Sectional Championship, Morgan toed the line for the 1500 meter. The pistol sounded and the runners charged into the first turn. The plan was to position herself near the back of the front pack and from there monitor and move. For 400 meters, the plan was working, but in the next two laps, things went south. For no apparent reason, Morgan slowed. Runner after runner passed by while I alternately screamed at her and muttered to myself, wondering what was wrong as she sank out of the top ten runners, heading straight for the big disappointment.

They passed the 800 meter mark. I was already mentally preparing her race post-mortem when she began moving. It was nothing dramatic, hinted at only by a subtle shift in body posture. But she was driving, clocking her third 400 meter--usually the slowest of the race--four seconds faster than her second. While others flagged, Morgan moved up places, checking off competitors one-by-one, like items on a to-do list. It was a long way to come back, but by the final lap and a half, she had moved within striking distance of the leaders. Calmly, she dialed up a strategic surge to close on the front runners, and her finish sprint saw her powering away from the field to claim the 1500 meter championship.

I stood trackside, shaking my head in disbelief as she sauntered over from the finish line, a wide smirk stretching her face. "I had you worried, didn't I?" she said.

***

I was on my second turn at Steve Magness's book, *The Science of Running*, and the next section for the morning's read was titled 'Stress and Recovery.'

How fortuitous. We had three practice days before the SCAC Championship. If you subtracted the pre-day, scheduled as a light activation of the systems and baton drills for relay squads, that left only two practice sessions to consider. And 'consider' meant focusing on the runners. They had now been at it for two and a half months, that time filled with neighborhood roads and hills, tight and stuffy hallways, an occasionally melted track, and competitions, every day of that stretch instructive if you paid attention. In all that time, the weather had never improved, but in fits and starts the runners had. The week began, though, with smaller teams because a significant number of athletes had not qualified for the league championship. For those athletes, all the miles had come to an end.

The story of any scholastic track and field season in our geographical section is about its time-honored process of narrowing the team even as the stakes increase. Planned attrition. This isn't basketball. You don't walk out of the arena one last time as a team that either won or lost. At a point in this runners' winter sport, the fortunate earn the right to compete in the league championship. Others close the book on the season, satisfied or otherwise. The team shrinks. Then, after leagues, except for the relays a coach is allowed to fashion, only those who have met an individual sectional standard move on. The team shrinks again. Following sectionals, only athletes and relays meeting even harder standards advance to the Open Qualifier meet. A shot at making the state championship lies there. By then it's down to a tight group, the team's most talented. Smaller still. At the Open Qualifier, there are often fewer spectators up in the balcony because fewer parents have kids remaining in the hunt for mastery or winning. Even as the competitive stakes crescendo, the place is comparatively subdued. It's all business in determining the best the section will send to states. Though drama remains, a more workman-like attitude prevails. Gone are the raucous winter nights of athletes trying their best, getting it right or making mistakes in front of family and friends and teammates who fill the place with noise and hope. The whole body of the sport was on display then, but now all the athletes have polish and none are average. At the Open Qualifier, with some fanfare and a few surprises, the select few above-average athletes 'make states.' They are the best of the best--and compared to December meet rosters, for each team they are very few in number. Those athletes beam and exchange hi-fives with coaches when success means the achievement of an abstract: excellence. Their parents applaud from the balcony, and pictures will come later. The sport, again, has achieved its subtractions.

***

Sick and listless all night, I slept in our guest room to reduce the risk of giving whatever I had to my wife. Feeling slightly better when I woke and thankful for the retiree's ability to sleep in, I hoped this was some variation of those infrequent head colds that feel worse than they actually are. Outside—bitter cold again. Most of the schools were on a two-hour delay.

By 10:00 a.m., our fate was sealed. The area schools had all closed, West Genesee among them, and with all those cancellations disappeared the evening's SCAC Championship. Soon, a 'plan' was emailed to all the league representatives, one that would re-schedule the championship to Sunday, February 10th. At first I thought, what the hell, extend the season for some team members—no problem. But the problem, as one representative emailed to others was that it created a string of 3 meets in 7 days. No way could that work for athletes aiming at Open Qualifiers, our gateway to the state championship. Those qualified athletes would arrive at their most important meet of the year over-raced and fatigued. A coach could have held out all his or her best individuals from our re-scheduled league championship, but then what would have been the purpose of the SCAC championship, especially if it contested *after* our more important Sectional Championship? I considered the athletes who had worked hard to deserve chances to compete at the league championship, athletes without the qualifying standards to make Sectionals. Steve, Justin, Aidan and Jack were slated to race the 4x800 at leagues. They weren't our fastest four, but they had earned the opportunity with their seasonal efforts. Still, like other coaches, I could not compromise the possibilities for others by piling on meets or watering down championship rosters. So, when I was polled with the other representatives, I voted no to rescheduling. Then I went back to bed.

February

***

I was early to our third of the upper gym. Recent snow days had caused other sports cancellations--and with that had come a flurry of make-up dates. The gym was already prepped for a postponed basketball game. Fortunately, our janitors remembered us and had not pulled the end bleachers out and over our practice space. So, once our smaller championship crew arrived, I took visual attendance and discussed the afternoon.

The first order of business was to announce my unsuccessful appeal attempt to have Pam and Sandy qualified for the Sectional Championship in their individual event specialties. Both had come close, very close, to the event standards required. Sandy was .01 seconds off the 55 meter standard and Pam .55 seconds beyond the 1500 meter standard. Both had missed a final opportunity to meet their standard at our cancelled league championship, which was one of the points I made in their appeals—but to no avail. Both were disappointed, yet both still had the opportunity of racing relay events in the sectionals meet.

Steve, Justin, Aidan and Jack, our four league 4x800 guys, sat on the floor, waiting. I had emailed them the day after that canceled championship to say they would still need to be at practices because they were racing the 4x800 at Sectionals instead. Unexpectedly promoted to a bigger stage, they were pumped and nervous simultaneously.

For distance runners, the day would be a medium-intensity fartlek run in the neighborhood, and those four guys headed out

[84]

with the others while I considered what to do with MaryAnn. MaryAnn's personal best mark in the Weight Throw had made her the first Wildcat to ever qualify for sectionals in that event. What I could proficiently coach in the Weight Throw event would fit in a thimble, but I'd always made a habit to watch athlete movement patterns in various events, whether in person or on video. I was weak in throwers' proper movement physics and the drills to promote it, but I at least knew what the motions should look like. My former co-coach and our outdoor track throws expert, Coach Corley, had made a habit of periodically dropping in on our practices to briefly observe our throwers and then offer suggestions. The last time in, Coach had noticed MaryAnne releasing with too much weight on her left foot and thought a verbal cue and practice might help.

With no other throwers qualified for the championship and my distance crew out on their run while Coach P. worked the small squad of sprinters in the upstairs long hallway, MaryAnne and I worked 1-on-1 in our small third of the gym. The athletic director, setting up the basketball scorers table, watched casually as I reminded her to power more off the right and rear foot. She listened, tried, then tried again, working through the awkwardness of altering a habitual motion. Slowly, she began to feel more comfortable with it. Coach C.'s suggestion had worked, and MaryAnne finished the session in good spirits just as the distance crew returned, stripped off layers and headed to the oval for 4x200 meters.

The sharpening drill we regularly used at the end of hard days was intended to cement relaxation with velocities when tired. The fifteen seconds between one-lap circuits of our halls provided time for only a deep breath or two. The velocities themselves, especially with tight hallway corners, were slightly slower than the 200 meter average for their 800 meter personal records.

There are various and psychologically proven rationales for these kinds of 'add-on' pieces to a middle-distance runner's day. The all-out 400 meter 'added' to some of our indoor hallways sessions of intervals is another example. Our "7 seconds" hill drills in cross-country is yet another. Sometimes, a day's finale is just the strides or sprints that, after a fashion, are felt necessary to 'complete the day' for our athletes, as though walking off without them would leave their day's efforts incomplete. What I always appreciated as much about the drills, though, was the attitude of the runners, already fatigued, stepping to the line without complaint.

"15 seconds?" someone asked, checking about the recoveries.

"Yup, 15 seconds."

Around the hallways they zipped.

***

After our short bus ride to the OCC track for the sectional championship, and after settling in our small boys/girls' teams and checking off the Leonetiming entry lists, there was a little time to lean against the timing area rail with an old coaching colleague and chew the fat. This was still our season with no officials, still on strike, and so it took only a short time to get around to that. Thanks to everyone pitching in, we had just about made it through the competitive schedule without major problems—and everyone now knew we would make it. Most of the athletes had hardly noticed the difference, but you couldn't count many coaches happy about the ordeal--and most had an opinion. "There is another side to this," one of the officials I knew had told me a few days earlier. "I am sure there is," I had answered, "but we haven't heard it, and our side of the story isn't very flattering to you guys." I mentioned that to my colleague, and then I groused with other coaches about my lost athlete appeals. Soon enough, though, runners veered off the track and hats were removed. Coach Jenson boomed the national anthem in his resonant baritone, and the championship was underway.

Never as good as you want, but never as bad as feared either—that's pretty much the reality of affairs involving large numbers of young adults. Track meets follow that unofficial rule. Preach health and sleep and nutrition in the lead up to an important competition, and someone will get sick the day before. You can bank on it. Some celestial law of balance is always at play. So, when Runner T's elaborate race plan went to hell a little over halfway into his race, and I could see he had no useful Plan B, I became a respectful witness to T's disappointment—and a quiet one, too. Track-side screaming each lap around would change exactly nothing. Instead, I spent time wondering what T would offer post-race about his effort. Maybe he would offer a tidbit of truth that, even if not soothing at the moment, might later provide some useful insight for his Race Analysis and better efforts in the future. That was, after all, the process we preached.

Near meet's end, our sectionals neophytes queued on the start line, then three stepped back to their wait zone and left Steve alone, gripping the baton and staring ahead intently. With the gun, adrenalin got the better of him as he jumped his first two laps, racing only two tenths slower than his all-time PR at the 400meter distance. Then he slammed into the physiological wall hard. All his systems were probably screaming *help*! as he decelerated in the second half of his leg. He fought it, though, and struggled into the exchange zone with an amazing five second PR. The handoff went free of theatrics. "Nice," I congratulated him as we watched Justin circle with similar over-enthusiasm. When Justin wobbled from the track, and Aidan hummed off around the first turn, I gave Justin his split, a 6.3 second all-time PR. "Two for two," I announced. The goal, they'd been told, was four PR's to end the season. A relay time and a place would be, more or less, a matter of secondary concern. Aidan, pumping for all he was worth, raced the most balanced leg and came across with a five second PR. "Three for three. We need one more," I told my growing group of cheerleaders. And on cue, Jack came through with the slimmest of PR's, a 1.3 second effort, but a PR nonetheless. They stood around with tired smiles, exchanging congratulations. "And," I said, reminding them of their 6th place, "you just scored for the team at sectionals."

Coach P. and I stood by the finish area, armed with stop watches and hopes. It was the final track event, the 4x200 meter relay. We watched our boys foursome queuing in their paddock, waiting to be

[88]

called out onto to the start line. "I'm nervous," Coach confided. This was his same relay of seniors that, back in November, he predicted had a shot at the sectional championship, a school record and a shot at making the state championship. He looked at me standing quietly with my clipboard behind my back. "Do you get nervous?" I thought about that. As the relays were brought onto the track and officials made a final check for schools and jewelry, I remembered my old colleague, Coach Delsole. He told me once that, in at least one respect, we were similar. Regardless of the ups and downs of team seasons, we always sought to have some individuals who were at least near the top of sectional performers in their event, who were, as he described it, "in the hunt." Training to put athletes in the hunt because you knew they belonged there—that was when I was most apprehensive, the most pensive, the most worried because that was when so much was under my control and, so, my responsibility. Having, for years, watched some high-wire performances go marvelously well and others go disastrously wrong, the one constant was the helplessness you experienced once your athletes were on the start line or runway--and thus actually beyond your control. You learn to live with that, maybe even appreciate it a little, like parents at graduation. "No," I finally told Coach P. "Nowadays, I get more nervous about getting to the point where you can get nervous."

Our lead runner walked out to his staggered start line, while the others took their place along the outside of the track to wait their turns. Ours were the underdogs to a strong Proctor team but confident enough to use that fact. Win outright or be pulled to a best time--maybe that state championship 2nd qualifier standard that would allow the section to send two relays. The hay was in the barn and there was everything to gain, but we were merely those spectators now.

The start gun barked, and Dan blasted his opening leg. Two relay members and less than forty-five seconds later, the event had become a two-team affair. We chased. Esaias' closing leg was one of his best, but not enough to catch Proctor. Still, our relay broke the old school record again, they closed on the 2nd qualifier standard and, because of our cancelled SCAC meet, those four racers hooting and exchanging fist-bumps with Coach P. would now be designated league champions. The Open Qualifier was a week away. They had one last chance to "make states."

***

I was standing on the low stone ledge of the full-length window across from Cafeteria II. The window looks out on our usually snow-covered track. Translucent February winter light was peeking in, as though curious. It seemed to consider the empty hall. In early December, such sunlight would have lit the faces of a noisy and garrulous bunch of athletes crowding our "L" hallway warm-up circuit, all of them excited for the season ahead. This day, though, the light and I waited for shrunken clusters of runners to pop in and out of view. We were down to ten athletes who had met the standards for our Open Qualifier meet coming up in three days. Pam, Cindy, Tammi, our four boys 4x800'ers and others were gone, done for the season, but the ten remaining would reappear, pass, then vanish just as quickly. The curious light might have been expecting ghosts but instead found these fleeting and talented survivors of a long, cold season. In a month, of course, the hall would again swell to bursting with early-March bodies imagining glory in the outdoor track season. At that moment, though, the empty slate ledge was quietly warmed by its curious late-winter visitor—a scene where you could imagine a cat napping.

Tom

They circled by me on their cramped "L" hallway warm-up loop. The chill winds of winter waited outside, already prepped and ready to go. With a general conditioning run through the neighborhoods on the agenda, Tom had begun lobbying. Each time he and his buddies slid by, the question was posed: "Short Quartz today Coach?"

I said nothing. The previous season, I'd made the mistake of abbreviating their residential 'Quartz Run' by a mile for one practice, and I'd been regretting it ever since. There were no slackers in this group, but they'd work an angle if one presented itself. Tom cruised by with a tucked-in smile. "Short Quartz Coach?"

'T-hop,' as they called him, was on a senior roll. Strengthening into the fall, he'd anchored the cross-country team to a NYS Federation Championship qualification and a top-10 state ranking in the tough Class AA grouping. Moving to indoor, and impatient with my seasonal race choreography, he set the school's Indoor Track record with his first crack at the 3200 meter. Then he stepped down the distance and upped the pace, doing his bit for the 4x1 Mile relay that managed to clock the state's fastest time going into the National Scholastic Championship for which they'd qualified. Another March road trip was in the offing, and they were loving the prospect.

There was nothing in the steely-grey weather outside to hint at what would happen next, no way to predict how Tom, in a momentary lapse of judgment, would agree to a pick-up basketball game on his rest day that weekend and, of course, severely sprain the left ankle. His season, and the high hopes of our national's relay, would end with his apologetic Sunday evening phone call, the call that always comes sooner or later to high school coaches because these are, after all, just high school kids.

At that oblivious wintry moment, however, the athletes were circling the halls, relaxed and jocular, thinking only minutes into their futures where, as far as they were concerned, all would always be right in the world. With his buddies, T-hop cruised past again and smiled in that mischievously sly manner of his.

"Short Quartz today Coach?"

***

All area schools this February day were out for the storm, ours included. Nothing actually happened until a light snow began falling about 8:45 a.m., but everyone knew what would follow. The upstate telephone chain of superintendents, west to east, had verified the storm would be a gob-smack of varied conditions, and no one was taking the chance of kids stranded at schools with frantic parents. Sure enough, the snow intensified steadily through the morning, calling in reinforcements. All day, it attacked. Snow turned to crystalline snow, and on a second time out to shovel the driveway, I muscled a thin but heavy layer, like the icing on my mother's Betty Crocker cakes. Then came ice pellets and, finally, a rain/snow mix. Tree limbs sagged under the weight. Roads clogged. Thankfully, this was a 'pre-day' before Wednesday's State Qualifier Meet, so little preparation was sacrificed to the storm. But would it linger overnight? Everyone waited and worried.

***

Early morning. A wide swath of Central New York schools were on a two-hour delay. The major exception was the Syracuse City Schools, who had surrendered to snowy weather for a second day. Sunshine, though, streamed through my study window. The glittering mantle of white atop lawns and roofs was still, I knew, a crusted mess due to the snow-turned-rain of late last evening. I sipped my coffee, read and waited.

If enough school delays turn into cancellations, you reach the trigger-point for indoor track cancellations. At that percentage, which is 50% of schools lost to weather, any scheduled meet is postponed or cancelled. Our section's varied geography, though, creates curious circumstances. You can be soaking up sunshine in the southern hills of Section III while lake-effect blizzards engulf the middle or northern area schools. Sometimes a west-to-east storm on a southerly track creates the opposite effect, leaving northern schools unscathed. It doesn't matter. If half the schools are called out, the other half are out of luck too. For the regular-season invitationals, we accept that luck of the weather draw, and a cancelled meet stays cancelled. Our Section III Open Qualifier, however, is different. The coordinators usually manage to negotiate a snow-date in the event of any sectional championship or state qualifier postponement—or they simply scramble. Only the year before, snow had forced a state qualifier postponement to a hastily arranged Sunday date. So, from a formally scheduled family trip that morning, I left Toronto, Canada at 4:00 a.m. to return to our Syracuse SCR track. The late-night partiers had been singing and stumbling into our hotel as I drove off. We qualified a girls 4x400 relay for states that long day, and Easais made the 200 meter leg of the Intersectional Relay. I was foolish enough to believe I had paid my cancellation dues with that adventure, but sometimes karma is just a concept. The weather this day, however, was kind, and after scrapping and cleaning, our school opened withed most others.

Toward late morning, the e-mail arrived. *Hi Coach P., it's Jackie. I just wanted to let you know that yesterday I had a really painful headache and nasal congestion throughout the whole day and I couldn't sleep last night because the nasal congestion got worse as well as me feeling dizzy. I am visiting the doctor's office this morning and I will keep you updated and I'm hoping after I take some medicine everything will be fine because I know today is a very important race day and the last thing I want is to let our relay team down after all the hard work this season.*

I appreciated Jackie's resolve and sense of responsibility, but the reality was obvious; she would not be able to compete. To make matters worse, those not qualified for this meet had finished their seasons. We had not asked a relay alternate to train with no expectation of competing. I had rolled the dice—and lost. At school, Coach P. got to work while I contacted one of the sectional coordinators about our dilemma and petitioned to add an alternate even though entries were closed. In short order, permission was extended, and Coach P. alerted me that our only possible replacement had agreed, on short notice, to compete. Tammi would be on the bus that afternoon.

Tammi had never followed through on her wish expressed that cold December afternoon atop Monte Vista hill. She had not quit. Through the season, the flame of desire had neither flared nor been totally snuffed out. Her competitive results were desultory, but she gamely persevered, fueled not by the joys of middle-distance running but always aware of what her afternoon teammates meant to her. During those weeks and months, if I had, at odd moments, shaken my head at her considerable but squandered potential, I just as often reminded myself of what the sport had been able to provide her, which also seemed considerable. There was one thing, however, I could always count on—Tammi's implacable honesty with me. Good days, bad days, lost days—she was always willing to tell me which was which, even if she did not know why. And that mattered too—a lot. So here was Tammi once more, almost a week after her season had ended, willing to sub in at the last moment for her teammates.

Late in the morning, the headache and dizziness plaguing Jackie had been diagnosed as the flu, so that was that. When Tammi boarded the bus as her replacement, I thanked her publicly, in front of the others, and at 2:20 p.m., we pulled out.

We rocked down the Thruway, the white, blustery landscapes sliding by. "Well, now that we are halfway through February, it finally feels like deep winter," I told Coach P. "Yup," he agreed. Our third time to Utica this winter, the trip went easily, and when we emerged from the air-lock into the track, the team area was sparsely populated. This was an Open Qualifier, after all, with its shrunken field of the best of the best. The assumption I shared with Coach P. was that our best chance to advance athletes to states lay with the boys 4x200. Matt in the 1600, the girls 4x200 and Sandy in the 600 were dark horse possibilities—but they would at least have their chance.

Dan and Easais raced early in the 55 meter dash, finishing 5th and 6th in the finals. After sufficient time to rest and recover, they lined up with Pat and Jake for the 4x200 relay. The favored Proctor team stood aside them. I left Coach P. and walked to the 200 meter surge point in the backstretch where they would lean hard into their second and final curve. Coach wanted Esaias to race first so he could keep the team close to Proctor and in contention. That would place pressure on the following runners, but pressure was what the meet was all about. Beat Proctor or race so close that they met the second qualifier state championship standard of 1:34.94--the goal was simple. Tactics

[96]

were limited. Sprint all-out all the way, and execute precise, clean baton hand-offs. Hundredths, perhaps tenths, of a second could be gained with precision hand-offs—they had heard that declaration ad nauseum from both Coach P. and myself.

Easias bolted out and powered by me down the backstretch. He gave the team the lead in the first leg, but we soon knew why. Proctor had also altered their typical order of runners. Their fastest relay member now came second, and he fired by Jake to open a small lead, which held through Pat's third leg. All the handoffs had gone well, and Dan took the baton, now staring out at Proctor's sizeable lead. He knew he was chasing the team's second-best option, the clock and the state standard for second qualifiers. Dan charged by me as I shouted support, then he roared around turn #2 and with a final push burst across the finish. The Utica track had no large linked scoreboard like the SRC facility, so I trotted across the infield where Coach and the others were huddled to watch times come up on the portable timer clock. When I arrived, it was all smiles and handshakes and backslaps. Their relay time flashed again: 1:34.75. What Coach P. in November had predicted was possible had become reality. Esaias, Jake, Pat and Dan were 'going states.'

The celebration was cut short by the girls 4x200 taking the track. I jogged again to the back straight just in time to watch catch Waverly whizzing by with a strong opening leg that put them in the hunt. Sandy followed before Tammi came churning around the first turn with arms pumping furiously, racing for all she was worth. She handed off to Tara, but by then it was clear they were racing for the chance to be racing together, which is never a bad reason. They placed 5th with a credible time. Tammi had done just fine and was properly pleased. Losing Jackie had hurt, but it did not cost them a trip to states. Four other teams were just that much better.

No scholastic coach is really all that precise at predicting their athletes' performances. But with experience, you can get close.

The training efforts that lead into a race, an athlete's body language on race day, their projected attitude—all those signals can be read and, based on the field, produce reasonable guesses about how they will perform. That assumes nobody falls or trips someone up. Most athletes develop an emotional M.O., and if you pay attention in your time together, you can eventually understand most of theirs. We had a runner once who spent a year dropping out of important races. A listless, unattached look in the eyes on meet days hinted at potential trouble. Then it only took a precipitating factor in the race—a specific sense of being out of position or being more tired than expected at a critical stage of the race. A wide-eyed look of fear mid-race was the signal that the end was near—and then she would drop out. Oddly, she always stepped away with me close by. I don't know why. I even went so far as to 'hide' during one race, leaving my assistant trackside for splits. So she dropped out near him. After a year of that, the problem simply went away. Another runner of another time seemed to carry his life's weather inside him as mood. Coach D. and I could read his body language the day of the meet, watch his warm-up and then-and-there make our predictions of a good day or disaster. We were seldom wrong.

Sandy, though, was not like that. What was happening inside on race day and then on the start line seldom evidenced itself. Practices were insular also. We knew what to expect—all out efforts, with Sandy often down on all fours after a particularly tough interval workout. Her M.O. was simple—full bore. That invisibility of projected affect before races was balanced by the stone-cold assurance that she would never back down from a race, she would never quit on herself, and no one would hear her offer any excuses. She was a dream competitor in that way, someone who rightly deserved nothing except more talent to match her fierce determination.

At the gun for her 600 meter event, Sandy was immediately caught in competitor traffic around turn #1 as runners jostled for positions. Instead of establishing a safe first lap spot, one that would prevent her from over-extending herself early, she was forced to move outside to avoid being boxed in, to swing wide. The race plan went out the window almost immediately, and I watched her work too hard through the first two hundred meters. We both knew what that meant. We had talked energy systems a lot, and her training had been targeted toward avoiding burning through fast-twitch muscle energy too soon. But circumstances had forced exactly that, and though Sandy attempted to re-group and smooth herself out in the second lap, the damage was done. That perfectly raced 600m of hers back in January, where laps times only gradually diminished in a controlled effort, the race that qualified her for this opportunity--that kind of race was now impossible. She pushed on gamely but labored to the finish line, last in the field.

I had no time to be with her, though. The boys 1600 meter field, Matt's event, was already walking up the track toward the start line. I scanned the row of talented competitors. Matt was not among them. Incredulous, I scanned again. No Matt. As the runners queued, my eyes darted across the infield, then down to the clerking table. He was nowhere to be seen. The official lined up the racers; the starter raised his pistol, fired, and they were off. Abandoning the race, I walked across the track and soon spotted him, perplexed, standing near the clerking table as the racers circled through their third lap. My look and body language must have said enough. "I didn't realize the time," he muttered sheepishly. I was at a loss for words. Once we settle athletes into a meet, they are responsible for monitoring their events, knowing when to warm-up, when to report to the meet clerk. There aren't enough coaches to shepherd all the athletes to their events. Veterans typically help the neophytes handle meets, but Matt, of course, was no neophyte. At that moment, I thought about the appropriate—or fair—response. His was a significant opportunity lost simply to inattention. Or was it something more unconscious and complex? I did not know and was never going to be told outright, regardless of how I framed the question. Coaches so often assume we are experts at knowing what makes these young athletes tick, what they want. But more often, we are only experts in knowing what we expect, what we want for them. So, I didn't ask. "Well, Matt," I said to him, shaking my head and leaving the sentence hanging. Then I turned and walked away. The boys 4x200, flush with excited anticipation, was headed to states. Matt's season had ended in a dramatically different fashion.

He never told me how he felt about that.

Coach Delsole - 2016-17

"Lou, I have to ask you a favor," I told Coach Delsole over the phone. It was this simple. With three weeks remaining before the opening of the 2016-17 Indoor Track season, I had no assistant coach. My right-hand man for the previous two seasons, Coach Corley, had early on told me he needed this year to supervise the winter lifting program for his varsity football players—and I understood his priorities. All October, I had offered the names of possible replacements to the A.D., but nothing had panned out. Whenever I stopped in for updates, the AD would just shake his head. Time was ticking away. A season of solo coaching was unacceptable; it would cut the program at the knees and cheat athletes, but now it loomed. For over a decade, Coach D. and I had guided sports together in all three seasons, but he'd retired the previous year because he had other growing interests and insisted those would interfere with what the athletes deserved, which was his undivided attention. He believed multi-tasking was for people who couldn't make choices. "Lou, I'm out of options," I told him anyway. After a long pause, he said, "Alright," and I smiled to myself.

We plunged into the season. Fourteen inches of snow decided to cancel our opening day, but by the next morning the area schools had dug themselves out, and that afternoon the athletes spread themselves on our gym floor listening to my first-day speech on effort, on commitment and on simply showing up. Coach D. didn't say anything to anybody. He just stood off to the side of the assembled montage of hopefuls, sizing them up.

The November snows melted into December days of clouds and chills. On one of those milder practice days, I brought the distance group back into the high school after a successful interval workout on the neighborhood roads. Our workday had been as good as Coach's indoor practice with sprinters was bad. Coach had already stretched out his squad and sent them home. He was steaming, but he wasn't ticked at his sprinters. The hallway he was trying to use for their workout had been clogged with out-of-season athletes, all doing their intramural program things, the theory being that off-season work would give them the edge when their future seasons arrived. We didn't see the edge. All we saw were talented athletes who should have been successful indoor track athletes taking up space in the weight room or obstructing the hallways so our athletes had to bob and weave around them, compromising our workouts. Coach had counted three different out-of-season programs that afternoon. Frowning, he leaned against the folded bleachers and watched me circle the distance runners for core drills. I walked over, gave him the raised eyebrow and got the unvarnished opinion. "Why don't we just forget about winter sports and let everyone do intramurals?" he spit out sarcastically, shaking his head.

The holiday calendar—and cooler weather--bore down on us, but we caught a mini-break when the temperatures inched up slightly a few days after the winter solstice. "Odd that 40 degrees feels so balmy," Coach noted as we drove to The Rise to meet the arriving athletes. Our tilted neighborhood road was going to host one of our group practices, an arrangement where sprinters, distance runners and even throwers would differentiate interval lengths and total volumes, but otherwise share the same workout. Much as anything, those sessions were borne of a lack of coaches to be in 3-4 different places—although we had come to know that the athletes in their own way appreciated those "Happy Family" workouts.

The groups quickly transformed the road into a conveyor belt of athletes charging up the slant, crossing over and jogging back down. Coach and I stood at our vantage point a third of the way up, watching and periodically playing traffic cop as afternoon elementary buses pulled in and out of the side streets, their young passengers with faces smeared to the windows, wide-eyed or waving. Coach had had his eye on one of his veteran sprinters for a couple of days and was annoyed by her lackadaisical efforts and refusal to push herself with the faster runners where she belonged. Watching her dumb-down the intervals just irritated him. "She's lazy," he concluded, and turned his attention to others. The runners kept circling. A girl emerged from a nearby house to walk her boxer puppy around the yard. It repeatedly leaped to the end of its leash, overwhelmed with the joy of so many humans passing by. Coach, of course, walked over to pet it, and the excitement was simply too much. The dog jumped, paws up, onto Coach and peed on his running shoes.

January came, and it was thick with hard workouts, our invitational meets and changeable weather. Storms blew in and out, lake-effect snow piling deep, melting down to a dirty gray, then redecorating itself with the next storm. I sent the distance runners out into all of it. Coach D's sprinters sometimes joined us on The Rise or at the Monte Vista hill, but just as often they bore down in the high school hallways, running the apex of tight turns on the downstairs 200 meter oval or sprinting the long upstairs hall with the 20-10-30-5 workout Coach had borrowed from his days at nearby Skaneateles High School.

Late in the month, after our final invitational, the teams grew smaller, with only top athletes continuing for the league championship. We entered

February, the coldest month, with less than a third of our original numbers. Coach made suggestions for the league championship roster, which led to a 4x400 relay that included two distance runners and two sprinters, one of them the "lazy" girl who'd since redeemed herself in coach's eyes. They raced to a league championship in school record time. A week later at the Sectional Championship, though, a talented Fayetteville-Manlius relay returned the favor, relegating our Wildcats to 2nd place--and then did the same in the 4x800 for good measure. We reduced our teams further, to just twelve athletes who had met the standards for the State Championship Qualifier meet coming up. The snow-storms returned to remind us they were not finished.

That season, I was always mindful of living on borrowed time with Coach. Coming out of retirement had been a favor to me—and to the athletes. He had been something of a traveled coach. He came to West Genesee after several years at Nottingham High School in the city of Syracuse. Then he left for stints at Skaneateles and Baldwinsville High Schools before returning to the Wildcats, where we spent a number of 3-season years coaching together--not enough by my reckoning. There were those who could find Coach's manner gruff, but I always preferred to consider him plainspoken and truthful. That manner, though, sometimes put him at odds with administrators or other coaches. Speaking truth to power probably cost him one of those earlier coaching jobs when he too plainly defended a troubled athlete in one district. Ironically, that straight-ahead honesty was one of the reasons his athletes—the ones invested in the sport—loved him. That, and the fact that he was funny. The athletes loved his jokes, even the second or third time around. And our wry take on young adults was similar. Once, when we stood on a track infield, laughing about some athlete faux pas or another, a fellow coach came up and wanted to know why we always seemed to be having so much fun. Neither of us had an answer to that. We hadn't really thought about it.

On the morning of our sectional state qualifier meet, my first inkling of disaster came with a glance out the window. Snow was falling as a slurpy mess in near-freezing temperatures. Storm warnings ticked across a weather banner on the top of my computer monitor. By noon, however, the snow had ceased, and an ominous cloud cover began to thin and lighten. It appeared we were in the clear.

But an hour later, the A.D. secretary called to tell me the meet had been postponed. "But I see blue sky," I protested. Then I asked the most important question. "When?" She told me the meet had been shifted from Wednesday to Saturday, and it had been moved from our Onondaga

Community College site fifty miles down the Thruway to Utica College's Hutton Sports Center--AND it wouldn't start until 6:30 at night. I gulped. That Saturday I was supposed to be in Chapel Hill, North Carolina with my wife, celebrating her birthday with her sister and husband and other family members. The plans had been finalized in late November, the plane tickets bought. In my thirty-one years of coaching, I had missed a total of one meet, that due to a family wedding. My wife, when she heard, was resigned. "Well, you're going to do what you're going to do," she said, barely looking up from the couch. And she was right. The next day I explained to the A.D. why I would miss the meet, that I would give the chores to Coach D. Then I called Coach. He was unfazed. "You don't have to worry about it," he told me, which I already knew. That wasn't the point.

Late that Saturday afternoon, Coach texted the team bus was on the way to Utica, and when I sat down to a gregarious family dinner a few hours later, I was fidgety. Six hundred miles away, four members of the 4x400 relay were stepping onto the track for an opportunity to advance to the State Championship while I was passing the table salt. Under that table, on my phone, I glanced at the Coach's text updates with each race. The girls won their 4x400 with another school record time, and all I could do was smile and ask for seconds on the potatoes. A few minutes later, I snuck a break and called Coach. The boys 4x400, not expected to win and without one of their best runners, had nevertheless raced a seasonal record on the backs of three personal-best times. Not good enough to win, but very good. Nervous, I asked if the athletes remaining in individual events were cooling down and resting properly. I heard a quick laugh. "They're all business coach," he said in a matter-of-fact tone. By the end of our dinner--and the meet--four individual Wildcats and one relay had qualified for the state championship.

My day ended at the kitchen table of my in-law's darkened house. The others had gone up to bed. I sat in a small refuge of light, finishing our meet-sheet with long-distance data gleaned from Leonetiming.com. Coach D. had just called from a near-empty team bus that was rolling the night westward on the N.Y. Thruway, nearing home. He was tired, but he had excitedly related, lap by lap, Carly's win in the 600 meter, reminding me I'd missed one of the greatest nights of all our seasons together. "You would have loved it, coach," he said, his voice rising as he described Carly simply powering away from all challengers in the final lap of her race. "On that last lap, she just dropped the hammer."

Spring

"There are no dress rehearsals."
—Ted Levy

The clouds spoke first. The day had belonged to them, so when the runners arced the road's curve along the creek, it was the clouds that graciously stepped aside and allowed the afternoon light to pass through. The light ricocheted around the runners, sparkled the raindrops hanging from field grasses nearby. The clouds, quiet at last, had no comment. They would have other days in a wet spring. As the runners climbed the first hill, some of them pulled down ballcap visors against the sudden slant of light. Others just smiled and squinted on their way.

March

***

On the first day of the Outdoor Track season, those once-quiet hallways of our "L" warm-up circuit had, indeed, filled back up. Girls track athletes, coming and going, stuffed the narrow confines. Spring was still three weeks off, and outside the looming plate-glass windows that team members passed, the predominate mood of winter continued--21° cold, winds gusting to twenty, a light snow slowly petering to forlorn clouds. The afternoon hallway silences of late February, though, were long gone, replaced by the crowded bustle, the noise, and the high intent of team members getting a first crack at spring sports.

I stood on the low window ledge and watched the masses circle. Familiar faces mixed with strangers. I looked for clues in the passing crowd. Who impatiently wove past slower runners? Who jogged contentedly, more interested in the conversation at hand than warming at the correct pace? Who was tall and light on her feet-- possibly a high jumper? Who clomped heels or shuffled as though unsure of anything except being there. Who, in fact, might soon become a phantom, one of the ghosts dissolving in the days ahead without a word or email? Was there anything in the postures or faces of such destined strangers that signaled imminent departure, or were those neophyte expressions merely the surprise of effort after too much of nothing all winter? There was a lot to take in with this first-day parade, but if some of the passing hopefuls thought our inaugural warm-up on the "L" was just a throw-away first-day introduction to the system, an anonymous primer on the procedures of the day, then those team members were mistaken. They were already being analyzed, sized up.

Cindy came by, gabbing merrily with a partner, eyes lit, face expressive. True to past form, she had waited until the last days before signing up. Cindy wasn't alone in dawdling; a few of my veterans had made an annual tradition of procrastination. But as the sign-up days had dwindled in late February, I had wondered if she completed her first Indoor Track season and decided this running thing was just too hard, its rewards too vague and too distant to justify the daily discomforts, the pain. Every year, potentially superior athletes had drawn just that conclusion and lengthened what Coach Delsole once called our Who-Might-Have-Been list. Cindy, though, had been one who made it. Her presence would create more depth on the girls middle-distance squad. She might also, I hoped, develop into an important cross-country team member in the Fall and strengthen that program as well. A convert here, a joiner there--in a school dominated by the popular 'rectangle sports' of football and lacrosse, runner-by-runner has been the only method for building competitive teams. I watched Cindy pass merrily by again and allowed myself some optimism.

Terri was striding through. She, too, had passed her inaugural indoor track test as a distance runner and decided to stick with it. There was promise in that stride, possibilities that, if liberated by desire, could result in a competent racer. My hopes rose further. Tammi was a few runner clumps back, locked in conversation with a buddy as she passed. The dad had already alerted me she would "miss some days" for counselling due to "family issues." I had assured the father we could work around her schedule. He was as perplexed as me, but we both wanted to believe a new season meant another chance at a fresh start.

Matt and Aidan, a floor below in the downstairs gym with the boys team, would have been two of the bob-and-weavers, picking their passing lanes like impatient motorists at rush hour. Both, with their fall and winter sacrifices, were poised for good spring seasons. They now belonged to Coach Corley, the boys head track coach, but would train with me. Matt and I had never held a postscript talk about his Indoor Track Open Qualifier faux pax. Sometimes, pressing an issue with a young athlete does more harm than good, sends the wrong message that the runner lacks insight or enough self-knowledge to resolve experiences or actions. I did not believe that of Matt. He could derive the ultimate value of his indoor mishap on his own. It might take time, but he could do that. A talk was unnecessary.

And then I spotted Lily and Jenna, my peas-in-a-pod 'walkers' from indoor track, now engulfed in the first-day crowd. They were moving a little faster this day, but only barely, a notch above shuffle. They still bore those disinterested looks, as though just passing the time while waiting for something fun to happen. I can wait too, I thought. And for a few days at least, with all the neophytes and naïve newbies figuring out this spring track thing, they would at least fit in.

***

The historical average high for this early March day was 40°, a nod toward approaching spring. But we never came close. In mid-afternoon, the winds gusted and pushed the 'feels like' down to 9°. That is the zone where the state's wind-chill advisory chart declares nobody is going outside to practice. So we trudged up to the our second floor labyrinth of halls and turns, our aptly named 'Grand Prix,' for an implausible indoor General Conditioning run.

Winter light suffused the block-glass windows where the athletes sat while I delivered a short lecture on building a large aerobic base of fitness, that base necessary for ultimate and maximum training gains. I drew two rough equilateral triangles on my clipboard paper, one with a larger base--and thus greater height--than the other. "You're all Egyptians building pyramids," I told them, leaving out the disagreeable historical facts. I pointed at the illustration. "If you create only a narrow aerobic base, the height of your pyramid will be shorter. That means later in the season you can't sustain as much of the harder training necessary for best performances. It will also be harder for you to recover quickly from quality days. So, for March at least, you'll be the Egyptians building those wide-based pyramids." Some heads nodded, those team members apparently willing to tackle the concept. Others, though, seemed mildly perplexed or even visibly indifferent to anything instructive after too many dulling hours behind school desks. "Yeah, I know," I said, "the Egyptian metaphor thing is corny, but it's true." The job in the weeks ahead would be to make some corny metaphor a physiological fact.

An indoor general conditioning run seems a contradiction in terms, but on more than one occasion, runners coursing our cozy Grand Prix course have made that contradiction work. The twists and turns, even as they interrupt proper pacing, serve as motivating distractions. And we had thirty-one runners, so the Grand Prix would be busy with bodies.

The janitors quickly noted our presence and tucked cleaning carts into hallway alcoves. The plan was to split their thirty minutes at general conditioning pace into two fifteen-minute blocks. The minute recovery between each block was mostly psychological. I held the only stopwatch. The runners would merely to count laps and listen for my whistle to stop and then calculate any fraction of a circuit. "I want you to feel yourself giving just a little more push to this kind of pace," I told them as they queued. They were ready—actually impatient—to get going, so I set them off in small groups. As they leaned left and disappeared into the back corridors, I walked down the long hall to my vantage point and checked the stopwatch.

Matt surged out strong again, ahead of the pack. But for the opening minutes, he was not alone. Peter, our 8th grader who had been selectively classified to compete on the varsity level, was trying to keep up. Not that he was expected to match paces. I had repeatedly told him he needed to train further back, with slower partners. "Train low, race high" was our mantra for such athletes who typically lacked the miles and the seasons to absorb hard work like the veterans. We deliberately hold them back in training so they did not injury themselves with enthusiasm and competitiveness. Then, once they got to the start line, we loosen the reins and let them have at it.

It's a strategy that has proven to work. But Peter wasn't used to following. He had won all his modified cross-country dual meets in the fall. He had finished third in two large invitational competitions, and at the season-ending modified league championship, he finished almost a half-minute ahead of the second-place runner. One of our coaching goals was to protect him from his own expectations, so when he wisely let Matt widen the gap and settled himself into more moderate pace, I relaxed too.

In and out of view they zoomed. As I barked out the accumulating minutes, they sorted themselves. Balancing pride against the dictated pace, Justin kept the young Turk, Peter, in sight as long as possible without overextending himself. Justin knew enough not to turn a GC run into a race. Behind Justin, a group of common paces had formed. Pam, Dan, Tammi, Lori and Steve collectively seemed to be feeling it, pushing a group effort that, for some of them, almost passed for a decent anaerobic threshold run. Going into a bend, their large group would stretch out like an accordion, then pull in tighter afterward. I let them be. Cindy belonged with them, but she had made a decision about the day and lagged alone behind--though she pressed on ahead of Erin who, having taken off the winter¬ for a small part in the school musical, was gamely regaining fitness. She bent herself into a slight forward lean, as though asking gravity for a favor.

Way back of them all pattered Terri, looking fatigued and lost in the endeavor even before the first fifteen-minute whistle. Her circuits were slow and obligatory, like factory hours being punched in. As she passed with choppy strides and a drawn-out gaze, it was difficult to gauge how far she had come as a distance runner. A harder judgement was how much further she was willing to go.

***

Lori, like a lot of others new to the sport, wasn't about to be rushed into middle-distance running. An affinity for the daily doses of fatigue and pain, for a kind of relative sports anonymity granted most runners, and for the need to regularly explain oneself to friends or family—those requirements are not quickly embraced. You can identify a potential for the sport in a lot of young adults. Detecting an individual inclination toward the demands of distance running dramatically narrows the field. Serious distance running is an acquired taste, and it's not, like other sports, something you can dabble in.

Unlike some others, though, who fail at other sports and try running as their last best chance at athletic mastery, Lori had talent. She went out for track the spring of her freshman year, and she did alright. I saw the potential, but it was her willingness to confront prolonged fatigue that captured my attention. That Fall as a sophomore, though, she was back with the marching band instead of on the cross-country trails. I tried. The following season of Indoor Track never happened for her either because she opted to sit in the orchestra pit of the winter school play. So almost a year had gone by since seeing her running.

The bitter cold of previous days had eased. By 3:30 p.m., when Lori and the rest of the distance squad queued at the base of our Monte Vista Drive hill, the mercury had soared to 30°, what almost qualified as spring-like. An afternoon of up-and-around intervals was on the agenda, so the runners poked their water bottles into roadside snowbanks, peeled off extra layers and waited for instructions on the day's training groups.

On good teams with depth, a lot of coaches use training groups like they would an assistant. Within those squads of joined efforts, teammates become the eyes. They also become the cheerleaders, the role models, and the enforcers. The harder charging, more established, groups will typically welcome a new group member, but they won't sugarcoat anything, neither the effort expected or the attitude required. You can add a new runner to that kind of training group, and by the end of a hard workout any in the group, if asked and if honest, will give you a rundown on the newbie's strengths, weaknesses and demeanor that will be as good as yours--or better. I have watched enthusiastic runners that I moved up into faster groups finish the day with a glean in their eyes, as though stepping shadow to sunlight where they discovered something new to themselves. I have also seen tentative or resistant runners spit out of a new group like a bad apple seed. So who trains where on those hard days are usually decisions with consequences.

Our experiments typically take place in the lower training groups, so those groups are more fluid and less defined, with runners moving between them based on the workload, who is out of school for the day, or who seems ready to move up. Back at the school, following drills, Cindy had lobbied for Erin as a duo partner. "Let me think about it and talk to you before we get started," I told her, wondering if I was in some sort of negotiation. Tandems in training usually work well with experienced and familiar runners, but in other instances they can backfire. Runners can make unconscious pacts. Two runners accountable only to each other can sometimes dumb down the work.

When I called out the groups, Cindy and Erin got part of their wish. I put them with two others of equal ability. That foursome could pace behind our faster front-running group of Tammi, Pam, Wendy and Lori. Cindy and Erin would, I hoped, pull the two others along faster and closer to the front-runners that they were all leery of pursuing. By May, it might be possible to merge the two into a large front-running group, one that could train together this season and in seasons ahead. That was the hope. But I did not count on Tammi deciding to reject her group's intended pace after the first interval and slip back to Cindy's slower foursome. I said nothing as Pam, Wendy and Lori ascended the hill without her.

All the runners quickly settled into their work--nine intervals up the Monte Vista steep section and then around the level top loop. The nine efforts were split into three sets, with a short recovery walk down the hill between each set. And we had visitors that day. The sister of Tim, our volunteer coach, was a community college student and, with an assistant, had set video equipment atop the hill. Our runners were to be part of a weekly YouTube presentation by the college that would air the following Wednesday. They had already recorded our team attendance in the cafeteria and the girls warm-up on "The L." All that remained was to gather footage of our distance group practicing and to interview Matt following his workout.

Initially, Peter again had expected to give Matt some company. He followed Matt closely around the circuit before they regrouped for the slow recovery jog back down the hill. I let him imagine. After the first set, though, I signaled him back to the chase group that included Justin, Aidan and a promising newcomer, Brandon. Train low, race high--Peter was where he belonged. But like a wandering refugee, he was soon outpacing those three and finishing intervals alone, standing with hands on hips, breathing deeply and waiting. Still, that arrangement was safer.

Pam, Wendy and Lori churned out their intervals. The three were well matched, though they stretched out in their finishes. On the final set, Lori surged in first every interval, where she would halt, wide-eyed, her body slightly tilted, sucking in oxygen. I would gave her a nod, silently acknowledging the change that was coming. Matt finished first and stood atop the hill, enjoying his interview as the others labored by in the background on their last circuits.

[116]

Slowly, all completed their work and wearily jogged down, then setting out for the high school for drills and stretches. Quiet seeped back in. I walked down for the drive back thinking the workout—and the week—had gone well. And the weather was changing, just in time. Soon enough, we would see 50° days. A planned "Shovel Day" on Tuesday with all the athletes would clear the track of its winter blanket.

Ron

Ron had had it with the weeks of taunting. A congenial guy, the constant lunchroom incriminations by another student that his was "a sissy sport," that distance running "was for losers," steadily worked their way up from his gut until one day, egged on again, Ron simply popped the bully-- laid him out lengthwise in the high school hallway with a 1-2 combination before an astonished audience of classmates.

Ron took his suspension stoically, and the first day back to track practice, he didn't wait. He walked up to me at the finish line, and before I even asked, he said, "I had to defend us, coach."

***

It's an unremarkable photograph of a typical March workout on our local roads. At first glance, you can see the winter snow has thinned and dirtied on the lawns--and much of the neighborhood has been rendered featureless by opaque afternoon sunlight strained through thick clouds. The trees are a blackened contrast to the shrinking snow, as though winter's darkness has seeped in and stained them permanently. The dry road taking up most of the frame is slightly tilted. From the top, where the camera looks down, the angle has been skewed by perspective, so there is an unintentional dishonesty to the scene presented. For the runners going up that tilt—my runners—it's harder than it looks. But it is obvious why I kept the photo. Some of those I take of our runners in practices, if capturing the right moment and the right place, tell stories beyond the day. This one is worth its thousand words.

Pam, Wendy and Lori are running almost shoulder to shoulder, a three-meter gap ahead of Cindy and her current soul-mate Erin, who is still gamely winning back fitness lost to her winter school play. Looking at the photo, the mind can easily compress all of them together and get to what it wants, the image of a training group, a confederacy of effort. If you ask any veteran coach who has tasted competitive success, you might be surprised to find his or her favorite remembered 'scenes' are not necessarily of finish line victories or championship plaques held high by smiling teammates. One of those special memories will most likely be similar to what's in this photo--an ordinary day but with an extraordinary view of athletes unified.

My old coaching assistant was likeminded about this. On better teams in more competitively accomplished years, Coach Delsole would sometimes notice a cadre of talented runners going hard at-- and with--each other in practice and interrupt me long enough to say, "Hey, look at that."

In the left of the photo, several scrambled groups slowly jog their recoveries back down the tilt to the start, and two figures have just begun their next interval up. But it's the group of girls that dominates the picture. Pam and Wendy are in sync. Their bent left legs are driving forward and through, in the middle of the support stage, shins nearly parallel to the road. A half-second beyond the photo, those knees will raise slightly higher as the lower legs lever out with a reflexive mechanics and the back foot of each of them arches up perpendicular to the road at the moment of 'toe-off.' Then, for a fraction of time, they will take flight. Running, in that instance, is counterintuitive. One seeks to control the amount of flight because "air time,' as they say, is slow time. That maxim, though, must be balanced against another, one also fixed in physiology and physics. The longer the foot stays on the ground, the longer the impact forces being stored in muscles, ligament and tendons for recoil force have a chance to dissipate. If that happens, too much stored energy available for propulsion in the next stride is simply lost. It's the game of just enough ground time, but not too little or too much, a Goldilocks moment. In those perfected moments lie the elements of an efficient stride.

Only small hints of their body form suggest potential problems. Both Pam and Wendy are leaning their heads slightly left, as though to counterbalance a slight tilt in their shoulders. That would suggest something's amiss in those hips. Is there a weakness there? They should be more erect, vertically true. Lori, beside them, is just that. If you balanced a level across the back of her shoulders, the bubble would be centered, no tilt. Even Erin, if you look closely, looks tired

[120]

but efficiently erect. Pam and Wendy wear beleaguered looks that contrast with the intensive stares of Lori and Erin. But what does that mean?

The picture reminds me that earlier, before beginning their rises, Pam and Wendy had bargained for fewer sets, for less work, or, as I saw it, less time in the uncomfortable state of fatigue that is the stuff of much distance running. Maybe their head tilts are just bad habits. Even if that is so, because of the structural symphony of the body's tendons, ligaments, muscles and bones that are entwined by the nervous system, tiny flaws will invariably diminish the mechanical efficiency of the runner, and he or she will wind up with less generated force and more 'air time.' Then things get harder. That person will be slower than his or her capabilities predict, less able to hold pace.

Maybe, though, I'm seeing something besides a bad habit or weak muscles. Volumes of studies describe the notions and declarations of body language, how postures message our true feelings, our actual intent, making a person an open book if someone is paying attention long enough to read the messages. Maybe that is true of running poses too. Maybe they are a kind of dynamic, outward sketch of the inner soul, a moving portrait of purpose. Pam and Wendy have been at this long enough to complete their pictures. Though the mood etched on their faces match the weather, there seems more to it than that. Some believe a quality stronger than replication or pixels attaches to pictures and images. Maybe the two of them are trying to signal something that should worry me.

Shovel Day arrived. Early in the morning, before shuffling into classes, many of the athletes had stored their home snow shovels in the custodians' closet next to the pool entrance. The custodians did not mind. It was an amusing diversion arranging rows of shovels they would never have to use. Following our afternoon attendance in Cafeteria II, a coterie of giggly girls approached me. To avoid a crossfire of simultaneous statements, I asked, "Who's the spokesperson here?"

"I am," Sandy announced, smiling, so I knew the request was not onerous. Sandy explained she was asking Dan, her senior boyfriend, to go with her to the Junior Prom. My job would be to distract him in the lower gym during our combined drills while she snuck in the announcement placard and balloons. Then he would turn, and there she'd be, holding an unabashed proposal in front of a large audience of accomplices.

"I can do that," I said, but then we turned to see the boys had already headed outside to shovel. There went the plan. "Listen," I suggested, "why don't you hide your stuff behind the bleachers and sneak it out after shoveling." Giggling again, they agreed.

By 4:00 p.m., our diligent boys and girls crews had nearly uncovered the track. Only a few snowballs and deliberately askew shovel tosses had found their marks during the work. While several boys distracted Dan, Sandy disappeared momentarily behind the bleachers. By 4:30 p.m., the teams had pushed off the last patches of white, and we'd reclaimed our oval from winter. Everyone posed near the start line for our annual 'Shovels-Up' group photograph. And Sandy, flushed and smiling broadly with the others, had her prom answer.

I walked onto the track early with my new long-handled shovel and a rake. High hopes suggested I would be able to turn over winter-compacted sand in the Long /Triple Jump pit. Then my small group of enthusiastic pole vaulters could perform pit drills, swing-throughs with drive knees held high. A two-step start extending out to six if the athletes could handle it. That would be a good first day in our luxurious 56° weather.

When I approached the pit, though, I noticed a splotch of snow at the take-off end. I stepped into the pit to have a look and my shoes sank into three inches of sand ooze. Stepping out and shaking off, I took the rake and tugged at the ooze, scrapping it back to reveal a lower level of rock-hard frozen sand. Science teachers could have trotted out students to marvel at this West Genesee version of the north Alaskan permafrost.

So we improvised. The infield grass was soft enough to absorb and hold the vault poles. The girls who assembled later in the workout were pensive, following instructions and asking the right questions as they swung into—and through—their short arcs, most with knees held high in the drive position. By the time we finished, the practice area was doted with the small indentations of knob holes. One of the girls, Tina, peppered me with questions. Had she performed the drill correctly? Had her knee been driven properly? Did I think she'd had a successful first lesson? Yes, I answered to all of them. After the lesson, she insisted on knowing if she could become a good vaulter. I told her it certainly looked that way. Two others came up and announced they weren't sure pole vault was for them. I said that was fine too.

My distance runners returned from their neighborhood Skyview run and set about the 200's I had prescribed to finish with a little speed. Most of the other training groups had gathered and gone, leaving just distance runners on the track. The girls launched out from the start line, and by the backstretch, it was Pam and Tammi striding together, outdistancing Terri, Erin and Sandy by a good 6-8 meters. I stood by the start with my arms folded and just watched. Lori was missing that day, not feeling well, but she would have been right up there with Pam and Tammi, all of them proving there is no substitute for developed strength and foot-speed. Successful middle-distance running is, in the end, a matter of accumulations, a massing of miles and of seasons. So much depends on a young adult's willingness to make time for—and to enjoy--those accumulations. I knew that, for the girls distance squad, there was no choice but to find a way to invest Tammi in herself, her teammates, and running. Even if others showed talent and skill, there was no substitute for her years and seasons, no one waiting in the wings capable to take over on a moment's notice. A squad without Tammi, either by her dumbing down the work or by outright absence, would simply be a subtraction.

Matt returned a little late, and as he jogged to the line to start his 200's, I asked him about that. He told me he had decided, coming back, to veer into the Quartz Way loop and lengthen his run.

Nodding approval, I asked, "Well, how'd that go?"

"Fine. It went fine," he said. "I just wanted a little more mileage, that's all."

I watched the Monday snowflakes, fat and lazy in the null winds, drift across the faces of our quickening distance runners on the track. So it was that from the time I'd walked into the high school a half hour earlier for team attendance, clouds had drifted in from the northwest and the partly sunny afternoon surrendered. But it was a listless snow, so we stuck with the plan, four sets of 2 x 800m at 5k pace separated within by a 200 meter jog and a 3-4 minute recovery between sets. It was that division into sets, I told them, that would allow most to manage sixty-four hundred meters of good aerobic work with power and form. "What you are looking for," I added, "is to feel relaxed at the speed. Not strained. Powerful but relaxed."

The snow intensified—or maybe the flakes just fattened. The runners churned air funnels through the slow swirls as they ran their eights, then collected snow on heads and shoulders as they slowed with their recoveries. The clouds thinned and the sky lightened a bit. The runners grumbled and launched out on another set. Then, as though pulling back a curtain, the sky cleared. They ran their final set in bright sunshine, even as the temperature dropped.

I directed the first finishers to put on jackets and record final set times. Assembled, I told them the day's finish would be fast. Eyes rolled, heads dropped, assuming an all-out, leg-numbing 400 meter. "Nah, this will be fun," I told them, sending groups to the other side of the track for a 200 meter blaster. One injured runner who was not practicing walked over to be starter for the small groups. They sped through the finish, and I clocked the time of each runner, then read them out as the next group queued across the track. The girls front group came in last. It had been an especially strong day for them, and Tammi powered home first in the blaster. As they stood in a small circle, hunched over with labored breaths, I read out their times. Tammi had already decided about the day. When she heard her time, she nodded, smiled, and announced to anyone who wanted to listen, "I'm proud of myself."

***

"Have a seat guys," I announced in the late March downstairs gym. Except for our small, circled distance runner group, the place was empty. We were a few minutes past five. David and Matt had just led the group through their no-nonsense, rapid version of side planks, leg-overs, push-ups, hydrants, and other drills. The runners had been forced to quickly shift from one exercise position to the next. They had decided to call it "Speed Core."

For our runners, core drills after a tough workout always felt like the proper final statement. I had noticed that the harder the workout, the better the core drills seemed to go, as though an exclamation point is being placed on the afternoon's effort, icing on the cake. David and Matt's barked instructions had reverberated through our empty gym, though that seemed normal too. More often than not, our small circle would be the last practice group to finish. The others—the sprinters, the throwers—would have wrapped things up and gone. We usually owned the echoes.

As they stretched out and reclined, I told them it had been a productive afternoon, a good Grunt Monday on the hills of Monte Vista. And it was. The sun had shone, the winds held themselves back and temperatures in the high 30's proved reasonable enough. They ran a repeat of that up-and-around workout completed a few weeks earlier. The times were similar, but they had attacked the hill with more intensity this time. Tammi, Pam, Wendy and Lori all closed faster in the third set of intervals. Watching them push the final hills, my mind had wandered ahead, across spring and summer and into fall, imagining the cross-country possibilities with this core group going hard at the season. "You should never think ahead to the next track season," Coach Delsole had warned me one winter when considering a runner's potential during the coming spring outdoor months. Then he added, with a twinkle in the eye, "but you can always talk cross-country." There had been no one to talk to on Monte Vista, so I had to imagine.

With the last of our group gathering running garb and offering their see-ya-coach goodbyes before disappearing, I sat alone in a folding chair at the phys. ed. teacher's table, listened to the gym's silence and thought some about future prospects. Then I silently warned myself. A half year—even two months—is a long time in teenager years. Young adults can too easily become the long shots at the end of a coach's dream. Then again, much of this sport begins with dreaming.

***

It is not uncommon to imagine track and field as something always living under a hot sun. Images of bodies sweat-glistened and athletes squinting into a hot sun between intervals is the norm. No one thinks about March before the grass greens; no one visualizes a summer sport in icy winds, sideways snow, drizzly cold or pounding torrents. Our runners, though, know March well because they live those days. Like it or lump it, they run with collars cinched up and protected by hats and gloves, waiting for the calendar to hurry up and deliver that first 60° afternoon which will be an instinctive cause for celebration. They race even as they wait, so we usually schedule a late March scrimmage with several other schools to nudge hope closer to reality.

By then, three weeks into the season, our young runners are understandably impatient. They want to get to the reason they came, so the timing for any form of competition is good, even if the weather is not. Race efforts against unfamiliar faces are a welcome change and a sign that the season, however meteorologically tenuous, is under way. Vanished snowbanks and dandelions then don't see so far off.

The first two years we held the scrimmage with just Coach Tuttle and his Skaneateles boys and girls teams coming over. Then Coach Rauber started bringing her Tully girls, and a few years later, Coach Reid began showing up with his Westhill athletes. The more the merrier was the thinking, and each year we laughed cynically at whatever weather arrived with them. Snow-covered infield or sunshine and melt—the athletes were just happy to be at it.

Nobody was arguing with the 50o temperatures and occasional wind gusts this year. The coaches met for a last check of the shortened schedule of events and to be reminded that one of the objectives was a quick meet. Athletes on and off the track would be given their performances, then be expected to report those to their coach or write them down on clipboards under the EZE-Up tent, as ours were instructed. I had again warned our sprinters and distance runners: "If you don't write your time down, then you never ran."

Coach Delsole, now retired, showed up as our 'guest starter.' As expected, he was efficient and kept things moving. He and I had taken over a few Modified meets in our years together when officials failed to show. The goal had always been a two-hour meet because contests drawn-out by slow officials, especially in upstate New York spring weather, only hamper the athletes. "I wonder if we could just hire him for all our home meets," Coach Tuttle remarked as Coach D. shuttled heat after heat of hundred-meter sprinters to their blocks and signaled ready to our timers on the finish line.

In our first distance event for the girls, the 1500m, a Tully runner bolted off the line. Brooke was destined to disappoint a lot of Section III runners who futilely chased her until she had finally graduated to a D1 college program. My distance runners had been warned and suffered no illusions as Brooke sped away from them. All except Wendy, who'd heard the speech but was nevertheless, well, Wendy, someone not afraid to put herself out there and worry about the rest later. She lasted at that furious pace for only three hundred meters and then fell back, but she was already well ahead of our other too-cautious runners. Brooke raced a scrimmage time unofficially under our school record, but Wendy raced the fastest West Genesee time of the day because the others were unable to close the gap she had originally opened on them. The standard advice to runners is don't go out too hard in a race and fade in the last lap. Good for her, I thought anyway.

[131]

Later, all the same girls lined up for the 800 meter. We had juggled the event order specifically to allow for that kind of double event by the athletes. Coach D. shot the gun, and I watched the racers arc out of turn one and down the backstretch. With a little experience—and by paying attention--you can quickly match what you see on the track to all those mentally-filed runner histories of practices, of their developed gait, even of personality. Already trailing, our front runners grouped together down the backstretch of the opening lap like birds bunched for safety on a rain-swept day. There was no Wendy boldness in this event. They all seemed to be reading their internal perceived effort and making cautionary first lap decisions. That was a mistake. The 800 meter, with a unique pace profile, denies anyone who races it correctly a late surge. Velocity diminishes throughout, so you know that the entire second lap will be a fight against diminishing speed and mounting fatigue. If you see someone excite the crowd with a heroic 800m sprint finish, it's just a neophyte or a dawdler who has logged a mediocre first-lap effort. For their cautious efforts, they lined up against the fence after the finish and waited for the official to announce their mediocre times.

At meet's end, we put two 4x400 relays on the start-line against three other competitor squads. Everyone was in good spirits, with first-meet efforts under the belt and the fifty-degree, rainless weather—almost spring-like. Coach P. had his four fastest sprinters ready to challenge our four best distance runners. Coach D. set them off. My distance runners typically love a four-hundred-meter opportunity to go all out, especially to end an agenda of longer races. They consider it "dessert," and most years they have managed to beat the sprinters who view all those meters as the marathon of their fast-twitch races. This year, though, was different. Waverly opened an eight meter gap on Tammi and the distance crew. The next two sprinters allowed the lead to shrink, but never disappear. Lori, straining for all she was worth, could not close the gap, and it was the sprinter's year for bragging rights.

Under that blanket of gloomy but still-dry clouds, athletes mingled on the infield or jogged their cool-down laps. The bleachers emptied of fans, and Coach D. chatted with former colleagues and some of our athletes. Then he wandered over to where I was tidying up the paperwork. As expected, he noted some newcomers with promise and was his usual blunt self about a few upperclassmen performances that did not impress him. I tapped my watch and twisted my arm to show him the time: 6:28 p.m. "Not bad," he said. "Just as fast as our moddie meets."

April

***

No joke. We went to bed Sunday with the bare grounds of winter-brown grass. We woke the first day of April under five inches of a white blanket. The early morning timing of the storm was particular in its effect. Our school called a 2-hour delay, so the students, perfectly agreeable, smiled and rolled over. When they finally boarded buses in late morning, the melt had begun. Unfortunately, that quick reprieve did not include our track. When I arrived at 2:30 p.m. for practice, the lanes were still effectively buried. Plan B. We switched the workout to The Rise on our neighborhood roads, and I introduced a variation. One set became two strong repeats up the 220 meter slant, but when they jogged down, properly tired, the third interval was a thousand meter loop around several streets at a slower pace, with a finish that came up the first third of our rise. The experts call that a blend workout.

At first, I thought I'd gone soft with the athletes in running only three sets instead of four. The runners soon proved me wrong. It was hard enough. Matt, of course, labored alone. No one could stay with him either on the Rise repeats or the long interval that completed each set. Aidan and Justin, though, gave it their best shots early on. Lori, Pam, Wendy, Tammi and Erin formed a tight group again, but the question of who wanted to lead, who wanted to be the locomotive that pulled the rest, remained. I watched them dig down around the final curve of each long interval and then muscle up the last meters to the finish, where they bent, gulping air. The day seemed a small step forward, though there were exceptions. Two of the boys—both newbies—declared problems. One complained of shin splint issues after a single set and was dispatched to the trainer back at the high school. Another asked to sit out the third set because, he explained, his knees were bothering him. I nodded and sent him back too.

There was no reason to doubt either. It is no easy task to get a handle on this distance running business, especially if the plan is no more visionary than to drop in for a season and see how things work out, or if the run-up to running has been couch-time all winter. For most of those folks, the results are predictable. The volume and the intensity and the mentality of it all, no matter how we try to portion it out, simply smacks them in the face. They get injured; they ask to switch training groups; some quit, hoping to find anything easier. Old story.

***

At 2:45 p.m., I stared out the high school hall window as snow flurries swirled across the track. By the 4:30 p.m. start of our opening meet, the temperature had lifted into the mid-forties—but it never rose higher as strong breezes lurked to thwap runners in the face every time they circled into the backstretch.

We were optimistic about the girls' team outcome in our opening league meet because the predicted matchups tilted in our favor. That optimism proved correct as the ladies won every event except the pole vault, where no one could reach opening height. They won easily, as did the boys.

Mid-meet, the girls 400 meter junior varsity event was stacked across the start line. There were no lanes assignments for this creative configuration that Coach Corley had dubbed the Waterfall 400. His invention was meant to put more athletes into meet events while avoiding the typical lane assignments of this long sprint that could easily add fifteen minutes to the meet. We had worked hard to make the Waterfall 400 legendary, and some of the guy's runners could always be counted on to hop on the start line, pound the chest and, just before the gun, hoot "Waterfall 400!" like testosterone-pumped ice plungers in Finland.

The girls' heat was quieter. Athletes stretched across the line elbow to elbow. The official readied his starter's pistol, but I motioned him to hold up. I saw Emma still standing on the infield grass in hoodie and sweats, unaware her race was poised to begin. I stepped over and quietly told her to pull off her sweats and step to the line.

She fumbled and tugged. I suggested she sit, so she did and wound up pulling off both her track flats with the sweats. The line waited, girls bouncing up and down in the chill winds. Emma, sweatpants and shoes off, began pulling on one shoe and tying it. She fumbled with a knot in the laces. The official secretly eyed me and made cheerful small talk with the girls still waiting and hopping in the chill air, some windmilling their arms. Emma pulled on the other shoe and tried to tie the laces, but one of the loops came undone. "That's good enough Emma," I said quietly, finishing for her. She straightened and stepped toward the track. "Alright, now take off your sweatshirt," I reminded her. The official had inched the girls down the start line, creating a space for Emma. She edged herself into lane one. The gun went off and they sprang from the line. Arms and legs splayed in a mass around the first turn of their Waterfall 400. Emma got out well enough, then she tired in the second 200 meter, coming in last. But she finished.

***

On the track infield, following a hard Monday training afternoon, I circulated among the T-shirted runners who were lounging a little, simply enjoying the warm sixty-two degree weather. Many wore the same look—a finished relief etched into a self-satisfied smirk, a nod to Maime Trotter's fictional line to Gilly Hopkins: "Nothing to make you happy like doing good on a tough job." Even those who had not mastered the afternoon's work at least felt the satisfaction of managing it. That was something. Their tough job had been to complete a "combi day," the marriage of different workouts consisting of two sets of Step-up 400's followed by a single set of 2-2-4.

The Step-up 400's part, far as I know, was the concoction of Coach Delsole and I, though we both understood similar workouts had certainly been tried by coaches elsewhere and in other times. Our variation arose from the notion of progressing strength-endurance and grit. First, you place a cone aside the start/finish line, then at 10 meters intervals further back on the track plop down two others. The runners begin at that furthest cone, run the first 400 meter at a designated pace, then, with a few breaths, "step up" to the second cone and run that one. Repeat the process for the third 400 meter lap and you have a set. Any dedicated runner can imagine the feeling on launching out on that third interval, especially if the previous two were strong. The pace, an important element, ranges anywhere from 1600m--or mile--pace to 5k. Three or four sets with 4-5 minutes recovery between each is usual, depending on fitness and desired training effect. Years ago, one group of guys completed five of them, just to prove a point. That was something to watch. Ironically, a lot of our runners pick Step-Up 400's as their favorite challenging workout, so we try to never disappoint them.

The 2-2-4 is a workout Coach D. brought over from his seasons with Coach Reed at Skaneateles High School. Like most of Coach Reed's training inventions, it's not for the cautious or faint-hearted. The 2 means a 200 meter at intensities anywhere from all-out to 800 meter pace. Then you rest in place 2-3 minutes, take off on another 200 meter, rest again, then fight mind and body in a 400 meter at 800 to mile pace. As with the Step-Ups, you usually go 3-4 sets for a full workout--and intensity matters. The longer 2-4 minute rest between intervals creates almost a repetition-type workout, but coming after two sets of Step-Ups in our hybrid combi session, I knew the recoveries would never be enough. The runners would be forcing additional muscle fibers to work when they'd rather be held in reserve, which was the goal. They would also have the splendid mental opportunity to practice pain management.

On this fine weather afternoon, Cindy still declined to join the front girls group and challenge herself. I decided not to force the issue and directed her to lead the girls second unit. Up front, Tammi, Pam, Wendy, Sandy and Erin would form their familiar pod, with both its promise and its potential problems. Cindy would fall in with Tara, Katie and Tammi. She would, I expected, pull them along.

Warm-ups and instructions complete, the front group had launched on their initial set of Step-up 400's, leaning into the first curve. I started a stop-watch--just to check. The chase group dawdled aside the track, but when they stepped on and went, I clicked on another stop-watch—just to check. Tara, a sophomore new to the team, hung with Cindy through the first 400, even as their group mates fell off. Gulping air, the two of them stepped up and into the second lap. Coming around, they gasped, stepped up again and drove the last 400 of their first set. Crossing together, they bent over, hands on knees, with identical time totals for the set. Once I saw their time, I double-checked it against the first group. Cindy and Tara had powered the first set twelve seconds faster than the front group. I smiled, gave them a nod and said nothing.

It was in their second and final set of step-ups that the cautious front group released the breaks. Body postures revealed the differences in experience, in developed strength and mental mindset. The veteran front group all finished faster than Cindy—though not by much—while Tara, with her lack of accumulated miles, had dropped off. She was learning some things. To run often enough to be good, to be better than average, there must be enjoyment in the pursuit's full range, from gliding along on an easy, clear-sky general run to the more robust sense of accomplishment following a hard day of hills or track intervals. Gaining fitness to the point where both extremes are rewarding also requires a certain amount of faith.

The runners rested briefly and then queued for their single set of 2-2-4. Warmer weather cumulus clouds drifted overhead, and afternoon sun played shadow games. I talked to the training groups about digging down, about finding the reserves of speed with willed effort. It was that typical exhortation stuff. They powered out hard on the first 200 meter. Cindy and Tara rallied, clocking the same times as their front-group counter parts. And on the final 400, even with accumulated fatigue, those two ran the fastest times.

So, following their cool down, as they were lounging in the grass before leaving, I had wandered over to congratulate them again on a solid day's work. I gave Cindy a fist-bump. "Impressive," was all I said, knowing she'd get the emailed workout sheet later that evening, with its set total times and its averages and its rankings of runners. She'd see herself at the top of the girls' list. Bright-eyed and smiling, Cindy mentioned the recent warm Spring weather. "It was so nice out yesterday," she said about her Sunday miles alone. "I was looking forward to my run, not just thinking about getting it done."

I tipped my hat to that.

Tiffany

For two years, Tiffany was a pain in the butt. Not so much for what she did, but for what she was capable of doing but didn't. Call it squandered potential. Instead of leading her sprint group in practices, she followed at the back end, a grimace contorting that pretty face. She complained her knees hurt, her ankles too, or that she was dehydrated and nauseous and had to bail on workouts. She insisted she was training as hard as possible, but who were we kidding? Meets followed suit, and mediocre seasons accumulated. A potentially talented athlete, Tiffany in those early years was, as she described herself in a senior-year English essay, "lusterless."

But things can change. Winter of her junior year, Tiffany was battling her personal Mt. Everest during indoor track: 4–6 in the high jump. Stalled at 4-4, all my physical and mental training techniques had failed to propel her two inches higher.

One evening at a late-season meet, I was talking with team members when my assistant, Coach Tarolli, interrupted me. "She's at 4-6," he said, pointing down to the floor where Tiffany nervously toed her start point. "It's her last attempt."

I watched Tiffany rock back and forth until the rhythm was right, accelerate down and around her J curve only to bail out on the jump just before the bar. She walked back to her start point, collected herself and took off again, bailing a second time. And then again. "Is that three times?" I asked to be sure.

"I think so," Coach said, slowly shaking his head.

I headed down in a hurry. By the time I reached Tiffany, the event official was shooting me a friendly evil eye and Tiffany was up to four. We both knew he was bending the time rules, so I calmed her, and she raced up and bailed again. The official came over. "Tiffany," I told her when he backed away, "he says you have to make an attempt or step out." She stubbornly toed the mark, zipped around the J and launched herself directly into the bar, knocking it halfway across the mat to end her indoor season.

Outdoor Track arrived that spring, and we rode the team bus to Fayetteville-Manlius for our first dual meet of the season. Opening against our division's strongest team was the luck of the draw. With four events on her agenda, we'd issued Tiffany her challenges. She got to work, placing second in the 100 meter dash while shuttling back and forth from attempts in the high jump--which she won with a personal record. Third on her work list was the triple jump. She jetted down the runway, stretching out on attempts with a light tap-tap of the feet, winning with another personal record. For her final event, she ran the second leg of the 4x100 relay, where she churned along the backstretch, opening a three-meter lead which her teammates never surrendered in capturing the win. Tiffany scored thirteen individual points for her teammates that meet, adding her relay team win for good measure.

In early afternoon, we boarded the team bus to take home an improbably 80-61 victory that would eventually lead to a league championship. The driver fired up the engine. Coach Delsole told the driver to hold on, then quieted the girls long enough to congratulate them on their victory. In a loud voice, he announced that this winning meet had been declared "Tiffany Day."

***

Early in the season, once I have sent my distance runners out onto the adjacent neighborhood roads for a general or a fartlek run, I usually drive the route at least once to check on them. With new runners who are unfit and unfamiliar with our routes, safety is the primary reason, but, especially with those neophytes, in the first weeks it pays to remind some that walking is not part of the training. The portraits of the faces I have discovered in pedestrian mode on the streets usually range from shock to fear, but a few had dared to project annoyance. All the neophytes have been reminded multiple times that they can, if necessary, back off a pace to keep running. They have our permission for that. But never to walk.

Still, some of those neophytes don't see it that way, and they often get support from parents or others who want to know what the big deal is if so-and-so has to walk a little. What's the harm? The kid is doing his or her best, they argue. It's only a sport, after all, it's only track. Appreciating the fundamental nature of the distance endeavor, then, its situated elements and its demands, usually takes time with the walkers--and some don't stick around long enough to learn. Fortunately, however, most do, and after they've heard the slow-down allowance repeated often enough, and after the veterans have modeled the correct attitude and behavior, I can stop playing detective and remain at the track to help the other coaches.

That afternoon I was needed. Coach Palmisano had planned time trials with his modified runners, and Coach O'Keefe was busy with her young sprinters, so I wound up helping the girls

[145]

modified distance group, about 10 in number, conduct their 800m time trial. Moving from my familiar varsity faces to spend time with "the squirrels" is always a treat, and one aspect of that enjoyment is how they are still so impressionable, how they listen to what you have to say. "Ladies," I told them before they got going on a final warm-up, "You are the toughest modified athletes there are." They particularly enjoyed that, though most of the talk was about how to prep for the 800m and then how to race it most effectively. Had I delivered those same directions to the varsity groups, some would have yawned, so it was refreshing to note the hard stares among these young hopefuls, the studious considerations of their best options to successfully race that difficult two lap distance.

I sent them sprinting across the infield and back to get the heartrates up. I explained the reason for that with the metaphor of avoiding 'red-lining' sedentary aerobic engines. Then I sent them a second time before arranging everyone on the line. Some hopped up and down nervously, glancing side to side. Others starred vacantly into the first turn, as though just discovering something out there. I instructed them how to step up to the curved waterfall start line with my given signal. Then I set them off, and within 150 meters I was asking Coach Palmisano standing nearby who the hell that was out in front by 10-12 meters. "Terry," he said, though I missed the last name. Terry was blasting the field, and her form was exciting to see in a young runner--smooth, functional, mechanically sound. She came around the first lap with a huge lead, and I said to Coach P., "Well, let's see what happens in lap two."

What happened, for a newbie, was predictable. She ran out of gas in the backstretch. The stride began pinching itself closed, and the arms begin to flail as she slowed. The modified cross-country leaders from the Fall season—Vivian and Greta—steadily gained on her, and by the time she labored across the finish with a contorted face, what had been an insurmountable lead was only a few meters, though she managed to hold those two off.

That rookie mistake mattered little. What mattered was that she had the functional tools and the basic footspeed, even if she lacked aerobic fitness—which could be developed. I congratulated her on the effort. "You could be a very, very good cross-country runner," I said, always thinking ahead to autumn. That's when she informed me she was a soccer player and then shuffled off. Greta, standing nearby, knew what I was thinking. She smiled. "We're working on her coach."

***

As we trudged toward the team buses to head home about 9:45 p.m., Coach Mercado asked me where this invitational meet ranked on my all-time list for lousy weather. I looked at our waterlogged, shivering athletes trudging across the school parking lot and at the rain which momentarily sparkled as it poured down through the stadium lights. "Right up there," I told him, "Maybe at the top."

It was windy when we arrived in late afternoon for the Friday evening meet. Though not raining, the meteorologists had made their promises, so I instructed the athletes to wedge our EZE-up into a tight corner under the stadium bleacher seats, and I used bungies and cord to lash it to the stand's support girders. With both boys and girls teams using the tent, the inside quickly became a disorganized mound of backpacks and bodies. I pulled on my rain pants and down jacket, stuffed gloves in the side pocket of my WG parka and headed out to the track. I thought I was ready for anything.

An hour later, the Chittenango Invitational began as just another blustery April challenge. Our 100hh event was a disappointment for both Riley and Carrie. No PR's for either, even with a backwind. Riley cleared the first hurdle poorly and never fully recovered. She lurched over the last one with all the finesse of a modified neophyte. Walking off the track, she was head down and in the dumps. Tara and Waverly performed a little better in the 100m, finishing 4th and 7th overall, but neither notched a PR. Then the rain arrived as promised, announcing itself first with just a few splattering drops, then steadily increasing in intensity. As the clouds darkened into dusk, Peter raced the rain, clocking a 4:58.65 in his Boys Mile, a time which that week would become the current #3 Mile time in the country for 8th graders, #2 in NYS. More importantly, his effort would also qualify him for the New Balance National Championship Boys Middle School Mile in the distant--and warmer--month of June.

By the time the girls' mile lined up, with Tammi and Erin in the 2nd faster heat, we were full into what the meteorologists had predicted. Through the wind-driven raindrops, Tammi ran conservatively, taking no chances, but she gained confidence into the third lap, and, as she was moving up, Erin was falling off. They changed places, with Tammi charging into the last lap while Erin struggled to hold pace. Tammi's reward was a 4th place finish while Erin faded to 8th. After, she sat dejected on a bench. Matt was working hard to console her, but I politely sent him away, gave Erin a light pat on the shoulder and left her alone to respect the moment.

The rain persisted, except for one odd moment when our girls 4x100 relay took the gun in the second of three heats and raced through a strange and momentary hiatus in the deluge. They won their heat and then watched as the heavens again opened on the third and fastest heat, slowing everyone. Our girls placed 2nd overall and met the State Qualifier meet standard with their best effort of the season.

Under their umbrellas, coaches peered at their cell phone weather radars, hoping for the break which would never arrive. Nobody was getting those best performances they had come for. Sandy and Jackie raced the 400 meter in a sideways storm, well off their bests. The lights came on. The elite Fleet Feet Mile was inserted at its planned 7:00 p.m. time and contested in the continuing downpour. Matt pushed himself into the thick of things but faded, finishing only 9th. Wendy and Pam placed 8th and 9th on the girls side. The rain pounded the athletes, with the only consolation a diminution of the winds.

Beyond 9:00 p.m., fans had begun retreating, and coaches

scratched athletes from late events. I balanced perseverance against absurdity and gave Lori the option of not racing her 3000 meter, the final event of the meet and probably still an hour and a half away. Shivering, she thanked me repeatedly and headed home with parents. Then I gave the 4x800 squad, the next to last event, the same option and received the same response. Coach Corley offered to have the boys team members strike the team tent, so while he monitored that sloppy task, I told the girls 4x400 relay, which was next, that they might as well race. They complained but completed striders on the infield to warm up. Then the meet official announced the boys and girls relays were being combined due to a lack of teams and in an attempt to speed up the meet. I gathered the girls again on the soggy infield. "Ladies," I told them with as much excitement as I could honestly muster. "You're going to win this!" Cold and sodden and resigned to their fate, they took to the track in a strange scene of desperate boys and girls teams spaced along the water mark under stadium lights in a rainstorm.

With the gun, the lead legs shot off the line. A few of the other girls' teams hung around for a lap or two, but after that our girls largely had the track to themselves, finishing ten seconds ahead of the nearest competitor. Sandy crossed the line with her slowest 400m split of the season, and the team logged a pedestrian time, but before they rushed off to grab packs and escape to the warmth of the team bus or parent cars, I insisted they group for a photo. What remains of that moment, besides memory, is the digital image of four soggy Wildcats standing in front of their stadium light shadows, pelted by rain, hands extended to grip the common baton. They are smiling like they'd just run away with the state championship.

May

***

No one was sorry to see April go. The weather, start to finish, had been awful for competitions, with only one decent race day. All the rest--league and invitational meets--had dished out cold temperatures or rain or wind--or all three. And this day's league meet at Cicero-North Syracuse promised more of the same. Not a good start to May. An upstate spring always seems, in the end, a roll of the dice. And like any trip to the casinos along the NY Thruway, you are just as likely as not to crap out.

Before attendance on the team bus, I knew of two who would not be aboard. Driving into the AD's office before practice the day before, I had spied Lily, shortly after school dismissal, wandering from a Dunkin Doughnuts sipping a large cup of something. She never showed up for practice. And if Lily was MIA, it was an easy bet that buddy Jenna would not make an appearance either, which is what happened. Both had also skipped out on a league dual meet the week before rather than deal with one of those raw weather days. Both had individual attendance averages under 80%. Neither had qualified for more than two meets the entire season. Enough was enough, so I scratched them off the meet roster. If either managed to make all our future practices, their last hurrah of the season would be our final league meet in a week. That was my final concession to indifference, and neither Coach P. nor I were holding our breath.

The boys and girls teams stuffed into three buses, wherever they fit, and we bussed north up I-81. The Cicero-North Syracuse and Nottingham coaches had agreed to a group Senior Day, so decorated poster-boards and balloons were taped to the stands and fences where parents leaned, camera's poised. Carnations stood at ready on the infield. Meanwhile, the sky hung heavy with clouds. One weather report stated 5:30 p.m. for the first drops; another suggested a reprieve until around six. The presentations of athletes went off without a hitch, and we hustled to get the meet going.

I had already projected the girls team scores with available athlete data. A win against Nottingham was expected, but the CNS squad we had lost to the previous year by a single point—that team this time around looked to dominate us. Coach and I had fiddled with the event line-ups as much as possible to create athlete matchups that might narrow the calculated margin. The rest, we had told the athletes, was up to them.

Toward meet's end, though, we were closer in the score against CNS than expected. The athletes had responded and brought their best. The girls had won several of the sprint events and held their own in the distance races. Unlikely to win the team score, their performances nevertheless were solid. And luckily, we had not been touched by a drop of rain.

As the final heat of the girls 200m sweep down the home straight, I stood with Pam and Cindy near the 3000m start on the track's far side. Their event was the next to last, and neither of their performances were going to change the eventual meet outcome from CNS's favor. Both knew they just needed to perform well, to take whatever competitive challenges came along in the seven and half laps left to their competitive afternoons. Pam did have an additional chore, which I had jokingly described to her earlier. "You tell Cindy when to take a deep breath before the start and just relax." My advice was no joke, though. Cindy had a penchant for terrifying herself with any competitive effort ahead, as though a little worry wasn't enough, as though she needed to rev up the heart further with trepidation. That ability to control inner drama is not an innate skill. If not inculcated early in life, it eventually requires practice. Cindy required a lot of practice. Still, they seemed fairly loose. Pam flashed me a casual smile as the 200m folks gathered their sweats and wandered away. Left behind was the small, brave cadre of middle-distance runners in the event, alone and separated from the bustle of the busier start-line across the infield.

The starter arrived to give instructions. With the girls 3000m and boys 3200m combined, and with their start lines on opposite sides of the track, he'd gun both groups off from the middle of the infield. A late arriving CNS girl swelled their group to four. "That's it?" the official asked with a raised eyebrow. "Well, it's not always the most popular event," I said, drawing wry smiles from the four now shivering nervously on the track. The starter went through the instructions they already knew by heart and trudged off.

"You just keep Pam as close as possible for as long as possible," I reminded Cindy. "Just work to keep the pace. You'll be fine." I patted her on the shoulder, unsure of how 'fine' she'd be after 5-6 laps. From the middle of the stadium, the starter blew his whistle to bring the two separated groups to their ready positions, paused, and then fired his starter's pistol. The runners charged off around their first turns.

One of the strongest CNS runners was competing, but she was doubling back, having raced the 1500 meter earlier in the meet. Distance runners typically find it more difficult to go from shorter to longer events. Physiologically—and perhaps mentally as well—long to short is preferable. And within the window of any meet's length, more recovery time between events usually leads to better efforts. Pam had raced the 4x800 relay earlier than the 1500m, so she had a least one advantage. I expected a battle.

The second CNS runner hung on for two laps near the front and then began to drop off, leaving Pam tucked in behind the CNS leader and Cindy working to stay close. I stood alone on my far side, watching and wondering. Every time they circled to the front straight and crossed the start/finish line, the official signaled the number of laps remaining. A small chorus of cheers and exhortations welled from the gathered athletes and parents in the stands but my far side was strangely quiet.

As they accumulated laps, dusk settled in, and the stadium lights came on. The rain had been distracted elsewhere, never arriving, and soft winds lilted lightly across the infield. The day seemed paused, as though to consider itself--although the runners could not afford that luxury. Dutifully, Pam dogged the CNS leader, riding her shoulder through the early laps. Every time she passed me, she heard the same message: *nice Pam, stay tight, you look good.* Several times, the CNS leader staged a slight surge, opening a 2-3 meter gap, but Pam just as quickly closed the gaps, as though the two were bungeed together. Cindy, not far back, had fought to stay near them, to give herself that chance.

Then they entered the fifth and sixth laps, that most dangerous zone of the race where fatigue seeps in and the finish line is still distant. During those long meters, the mind runs energy calculations and then issues warnings. Pam, the veteran, knew to expect those internal arguments and, aided by her competition, pushed on. Cindy, with neither of those to her advantage, lagged. A second off after four laps, in the fifth lap she lost three more to the inner voices. At the end of six, the differential between Cindy and Pam had swelled to seven and a half seconds.

But by then it was not Pam who Cindy was chasing. As those front three had passed with two and a half laps remaining, I shouted to Pam to go for it. And the Pam on the track at that moment, racing the darkness deepening outside the stadium lights—that was the Pam I had seen on a few special occasions. Normally, she was what others would consider a cautious racer, one who set limits on permissible pain. Where Cindy displayed a commendable naivete about plunging ahead toward the margins of fatigue and falter, Pam typically

[155]

approached that edge more cautiously. Some would describe that as experience and smart racing. I had always viewed it as something else, a limiting inclination. And my intuition had been confirmed on the few occasions when Pam had wanted a race result badly enough, and so ignored her self-imposed limits and took chances. Invariably, they were her best races, and she was running one of those now.

By the time the two circled onto the front stretch and approached their last full lap, Pam had passed the CNS runner. When they took the bell, Pam doubled down and surged out of turn one with a 15-20 meter lead. She charged into the back straightaway, aiming for where I stood alone at its far end. When she passed me, I shouted a simple, "Go!" The outcome was no longer in doubt.

Cindy, too, had summoned herself and gone. Her seventh lap had been four seconds faster than her sixth. She churned by a final time, fatigue less evident than resolve, in pursuit of second place. She had only two hundred meters to the finish, and she flew. Pam won the event by a good twenty meters, and although Cindy was unable to catch the CNS competitor, she closed. Hers was the fastest finish stretch of all three, and she clocked a time over a minute faster than her previous best during the Indoor season. I walked diagonally across the infield on my way to record split times for our final 4x400 relay. Pam and Cindy were trudging tiredly the other way to retrieve their sweats before a cool-down jog. Pam looked weary but satisfied, and I nodded my approval and offered a thumbs up. Cindy was her typical wide-eyed and buoyant self. "That wasn't as bad as I thought!" she exclaimed, smiling broadly.

"No," I said, offering a high-five. "That, actually, was terrific." They walked on, and I turned back toward the start-line as the official raised his gun and boomed to the relay runners tensed under stadium lights, "*On Your Marks!*"

Maria

Coach Delsole coined the nickname. He had watched all those seasons as I cajoled, yelled and demanded more from Maria. She was talented, but she was resistant. For Maria, pain had never been the challenge or the purifier, just something to be avoided. Over the course of eight running seasons, I had worked hard to make her escape from pain impossible--or at least less desirable--so our wordless disagreements were often. When pressed in practices to give more effort, Maria, more often than not, flashed a sour-puss grimace, her way of announcing exactly what she thought about this business of pushing through pain. One warm spring day, as the distance runners bent for breath between exhausting repetitions on the track, Coach Delsole meandered over from his sprinters group and leaned down near a weary, sulking Maria. With a mischievous grin, he asked, "What's up Pouty Face?"

Pouty Face hated running hard doubles at track meets. Her first event, raced fresh, typically went fine. She was, after all, talented. But then she'd tank in the second event with a JV-level result, heaving through the distance toward the finish line. At track or cross-country practices, she typically staked out a position in the group that followed the harder charging leaders—and then subtly worked to control her group's pace. One of Pouty Face's goals was obvious--to keep the effort levels out of the prolonged pain range. The other, which may have been unconscious or unplanned, was to wear her coaches down to acquiescence. It didn't matter which. The problem she had with the second goal was that her particular idea of stubborn kept butting against someone else's. Maria kept running doubles. Maria kept being moved up in training groups. Pouty Face kept grimacing. I didn't care.

Coaches are not psychics. They can never be sure what lies beneath the karmic surface of your average adolescent runner. Pay attention long enough, however, and you can make reasonable guesses. Her senior cross-country season, trailing the lead runners at the sectional championship, Maria came over the last rise of the 5k course and then simply blistered the remaining four hundred meters to the finish line, passing 3-4 other gifted runners to grab the final individual qualification for the state championship. She had tipped her hand, exposing that core of nascent toughness we suspected all along.

Later that school year, Maria was powering out of the final curve of her 400 meter event at the outdoor track sectional championship, trailing two competitors. She dug down, surged past one and went neck and neck with the sectional leader to the finish, where she lunged across the line, splattering herself on the track but winning by five one-hundredths. "Did that hurt?" I asked our new Sectional Champion after she pulled herself back onto the infield and we checked for abrasions. She gave me that sheepish grin. "Not too much." A few weeks later she stood on the State Championship podium with three teammates after they placed fourth in the 4x800, with Maria racing a critical second leg. Pouty Face had come full circle. She'd become a money runner.

I saw her after she moved on to run for Ithaca College. Our once-insistent 400/800 meter racer told me she had taken a liking to track 5k's. At the end of her junior year, her mother e-mailed me. "We thought you would get a kick out of hearing Maria ran back-to-back in the 10k and 5k at Liberty Leagues this weekend. She ran the 10k (for only the 2nd time and in the pounding rain) in 39:41, which qualifiers her for Regionals. She was seeded last and missed the podium by one. We were laughing today, saying Coach V. would have been proud."

But it was the summer before she left for college, I had received a letter. Maria wanted to thank me for all the seasons, all the pushing and the prodding. "You saw that I could do better when I didn't know I could." She also wrote that she believed running cross-country was one of the best decisions she'd been convinced to make. Then she added, "I'll miss fighting with you."

***

On a flawless spring training day, one in the low sixties, with lazily drifting clouds and slight breezes, Sandy and I had a discussion that--my fault--had waited too long. At the CNS meet the previous day, she had raced a desultory leg of the 4x800 and then logged a disappointing time in her favorite race distance, the 400m. Though her progress in that event had been steady through April, the increments of improvement were small, and she was running out of time for a seasonal goal, which was to be among the best in the section. The more important question to be answered was whether Sandy was also running out of seasonal potential for that event. After CNS, she had offered to run the 3000m in our final league meet to see if a theory of mine had any validity to it, the theory that a long-sprinter could, under special circumstances, have long-range promise in the middle distances. It was an optimistic theory, but with little science behind it.

Sandy had given up marching band her sophomore year to tackle the trails and longer miles of cross-country, but she did not crack the team's top-5 until her senior season. Work ethic and heart were never the issue. Physiology was. Short of a painful muscle biopsy, we would never know her general ratio of slow to fast twitch muscles, but workouts and race performances gave indications. We did know there were dangers in putting too many slow-twitch muscle training demands on a long-sprinter who depends on fast-twitch muscle speed. We knew how excessive or improperly applied distance training could erode sprint capabilities. But Sandy was a gamer, and both of us were searching the perfect race match for her persistence and her dedication and her fighting spirit. I put the kibosh on the 3000m simply because I considered what Coach Delsole, always bluntly on target with his observations, had told me after coming to watch one of our early meets. "Make her a 400 intermediate hurdler," he said.

Coach had some experience in the matter. Years before, he had trained Josh for that event. Josh was a quiet guy who talked with his feet. Without much of a thought, he had given up his Senior Ball to compete in the Loucks Games 400 meter hurdles because he wanted one of their impressively huge first place gold statutes. He came home with one. Then, in June, he won the state championship 400IH for good measure.

Sandy never got to witness Josh's relaxed, deceptive speed, but as a freshman she watched her junior teammate, Megan, pick up the 400 meter intermediate hurdles. Megan had already proven her mettle, racing a 200 meter leg on the Indoor Track team Sprint Medley Relay that finish 9th nationally. Her junior year, Megan raced the indoor track 300 meter and the 4x400 meter relay at the state championship. So that spring, when I told her the 400IH was "just a 400 meter with some things in the way," she laughed, got excited, and in June made the state championship in that event too. Like the fresh scent of spring flowers, the tangible proof of mastering the 400IH lingered in the air for Sandy, and she agreed to give it a shot.

The only problem, thanks to me, was that a mere four practice days remained before our final league meet against Henninger, her best chance to test the event before championships. So I gave her to Tara for the afternoon. Tara herself had been pressed into intermediate hurdle duties after Megan graduated because she was athletic and was good at all the speed-based events, from the 100-meter dash to the 400m—as well as high jumping. Tara dutifully gave the intermediate hurdles an honest go in the early season, racing it often, though the grueling event had never fully caught her fancy. I sensed she was perfectly content to hand over the reins to Sandy.

Tara started Sandy with elemental jumps over an intermediate-height hurdle set on the infield grass. I watched while supervising the pole vaulters. Sandy quickly mastered the basics, demonstrating that competence would be a matter of smoothing out lead and trail legs actions and then mastering the strides between hurdles. Despite her raw form, she charged aggressively at the hurdle, a primary requirement in that event. The comfortable afternoon was perfect for relaxed and steady instruction. After the grass practice, Tara and Sandy moved to the track and were joined by Carrie. They had set out the first three hurdles of the 1-lap event for run outs and to give Sandy her first experience linking hurdles at race speed. She would practice more of the same the next day, then the following Monday extend to five hurdles plus a 100 meter dash off the last hurdle. Tuesday would be for polishing what skills had developed in a very short span of time--and then her first attempt at the event on Wednesday.

I left the pole-vaulters to give the girls their starts and to observe. Sandy took off on her first attempt and misjudged her stride lengths, which cramped her up against the first hurdle. She stutter-stepped, launched herself and sailed over. After a stumble step coming down, she collected herself and churned to the second hurdle. She was forced to chop her steps at that one too and flew again, arms extending sideways like the main mast on a sailing ship. She plugged on and reached the third hurdle further out this time, reached for it and clipped the cross-bar with her trail leg, almost going down. Walking back across the infield grass to the start, she offered a pensive glance. "Not bad," I told her. "Try it again." Sandy toed the start line, nodding at something Tara quietly told her. As she settled into a start position, her gaze narrowed, and the face grew taut with intent. I knew this was going to work.

***

Tammi, you could argue, could never get on speaking terms with her runner's pain. There were other voices confusing those typical internal arguments any distance runner suffers, the ones that well up on the trails or track when the going gets tough. For Tammi, it was never just as simple as talking back to the homeostatic guardians, those messengers counselling her to slow down, take it easier. There were always those other voices, other litigates with their own demands, and that created a chorus of emotions: *You will never be good enough, no matter how hard you try --This can never be worth it, can never solve anything -- Any victory will be short-lived, so what's the point?* As a result, Tammi could never enjoy a clarity of purpose, a simple-minded desire such as laps run tired but fast. Too often, when pain came, those other voices insisted on being heard and being obeyed.

Mental mapping is what the scientists call our human ability to create internal images from real or recalled conditions, both inside and outside the body. Those images produced by the brain provoke reactions, some pleasing and some not. We call those reactions emotions, and they are private. Coaches are seldom privy to the full orchestration of conditions that provoke such reactions in athletes. What remained hidden for Tammi was the narrative behind her fear, the personal cinema of events, mundane or spectacular, by which she had finally arrived at a point where personal athletic challenges almost invariably signaled danger.

Most like to think that sports grant troubled athletes a temporary safe haven from whatever else bothers them, like confused birds coursing through sunlight in the still eye of a hurricane. But that's fantasy, what we want to believe. Most athletes, for better or for worse, bring their worlds to practice each afternoon. The notion of layered feelings describes how one primary sensation can provoke another. In our instance, a sports pain evokes images of other deep-seeded pains or sufferings. Immediate sports feelings, though temporary, link to more persistent and confusing ones. The best strategy to employ while things get sorted out, those athletes are sometimes counseled, is to avoid the discernable pain that provokes those other, more primary, ones. This is an understandable strategy, just not very useful advice for a distance runner, whose stock in trade is pain. Nonetheless, the girls 4x800 was on the line with a chance—most likely their last chance—to achieve the time standard for the State Qualifier Meet they wanted to race later in the month. Tammi needed to be a part of that, and she knew it, and she was already scared.

The teams of girls stood nervously behind the start line in their order of runners and listened to the official's final instructions. Then, the last three of each relay stepped off onto the infield, leaving the lead-off runners on the track. Pam would race the first leg. She hopped up and down and shook out her arms. With the official's call, all the runners took one step forward to the start line, crouched at ready, then shot off with the gun. The field closed quickly around the first turn, boxing Natalie in. She did not race her best split time, but she kept the team in the game, handing off only a meter behind the CNS leader. Wendy fought hard in her second leg, but when she passed the baton to Lori, the gap had widened to ten meters. With a traditional strategy, the third leg of the 4x800 is the slowest, but I had placed Lori there instead, who should have been the anchor leg. She pushed out quickly, closing the gap down the backstretch. With a strong second lap, she overtook the CNS race leader and was going to hand Tammi the squad's first lead of the race.

As Lori churned out of her final turn, Tammi stepped on the track to receive the baton. She shifted nervously, glancing forward, then looking back, feet trained to the proper start angle but nervously wanting to hop and twitch. I checked my watch and quickly ran the mental calculation. They were behind the qualifying time. "You have to go," I boomed to Tammi. Terrified, she turned to receive the baton, then bolted off.

Tammi ran for her life, clocking the fastest first lap of the squad and widening the team's lead. She passed the start line and geared into her final lap, eyes intent, arms tucked and driving. Along the backstretch, with the win secured but the needed time still in doubt, she bore down. Teammates cheered her through the final turn and down the front straight. With a final push, she crossed the line and wobbled to a stop, clutching the baton with hands on knees, gulping air. She looked to see me standing nearby. I gave her the thumbs up.

Tammi's relay teammates gathered with her on the infield, hugging, smiling, and congratulating each other's efforts. I walked over and gave them their split times. "You ladies are going to the State Qualifier."

Tammy took a deep breath. "Did you see me look at you when I came around the first time?"

"I certainly did," I told her as teammates nodded. "That was a gutsy second lap."

Tammi's eyes widened, balanced with the hint of a relieved smile. "I was scared!"

"Well," I said, "sometimes you just have to run scared."

***

One of the less acknowledged jobs of a coach is to see the future, to be able to explain to athletes the logical consequences of their actions—or lack of actions—well before they happen. We can usually portend those futures because we have coached through similar ones in the past. Nothing's a given, of course. Much in the lives of young adults is beyond accurate prediction--weather and desire, teenage distractions, and mountains of personal doubts. Experience dictates that we prepare the athletes to the best of our present ability and theirs. We strive to be fair and to be considerately honest. It is what athletes and their parents deserve.

The great irony of such guidelines is that conscientious coaches are often more adept at predicting failure than success. That odd juxtaposition, though no one's fault, balances on the fundamental ambiguity of sport, where it is often more about learning how to master failure than manage success. That distinction is important because, as an athlete, you are perpetually not good enough, always unfinished. One peak obtained, there are others higher. How you embrace that irreducible ambiguity as an athlete, to a large extent, determines your personal success. If sport was only about the destinations, sport would not exist.

So it was Monday, and Wendy was somewhere far away, probably lounging on a sunny beach in a warm clime, thinking about a run but never quite getting around to it. Her mother had emailed a notification weeks earlier, so her absence for eleven days while on a family trip had been no surprise. What did perplex me was how a particular parent could be so demanding for her daughter in a sport and then set that same daughter up for sports failure. I could understand the former; I was baffled by the latter. Wendy's 'break' could not have come at a worse time. Our last two meets and important preparations for the championship season ahead would occur without her. She would return the day before the league meet. Of course, I had her assurance of "staying in shape" while away, but that was a promise proven time and time again by other athletes, despite the best of intentions, to be an empty one. *Coach, I'm taking the season off this winter, but I'll be running on my own.* Or: *Coach, I'll be on Spring Break, but I will get in my miles.* There were only two guarantees with such absences—a diminution of skills and disappearing goals.

I could have warned Wendy and her parents of the probable consequences, but I knew the conversation would have accomplished nothing but more conflict. So I said nothing and imagined exactly how Wendy's season would end.

***

We started with the day itself. Spring had finally gifted us one of those meet days we imagined all of them to be: a western blue sky banished of clouds, a faint, pleasing breeze and temperatures poking above sixty. The athletes off the team bus walked with a jocular ease toward a place in the stadium seats of Sunnycrest Park. After settling their gear packs, some leaned back for a few moments before warm-ups, just soaking up sun.

Both boys and girls teams knew their greater depths of talent in most events predicted final wins on their league schedule. For the girls, that would mean a successful 5-3 league season, with only a final invitational and then the championship meets ahead. Track seasons, though, play out with multiple endings. A succession of winnowing's commences following the last league meet. Because the league championship allows a set number of team entries per event, the team depth chart decides who can be on that bus. In a typical year, half our athletes won't qualify to move on, and they know the end of league meets is their end too. Maybe some of those last-meet athletes welcomed the open afternoons ahead, but most wanted to move on.

Our erstwhile duo, Lily and Jenna, never waited for any coaching decisions. The day before, though both were in school, they skipped practice together. I could think of no response worth the time or the effort. Neither of them were resistant or reluctant. Even a low level of commitment would have given me something to work with. They were below even that. They were indifferent. They just didn't care. So I scratched them one last time from the roster and mentally bid them goodbye and good luck.

Pristine weather, the finality of the day for some, and the unpressured opportunity for others to go all out in preferred events— all those produced results. Sara raced one of her best times in winning the high hurdles. The team went 1-2-3 in the 100m. Matt raced all alone out front in the 1600m with a solid sectional time. He had won the New Hartford Invitational 1600m the previous weekend and was on a roll. Lori and Cindy ran personal bests with a 1-2 finish in the 1500m. Pam and Erin later achieved the same in the 800m.

Just past the mid-point of that sunny afternoon, helpers placed the 400 meter hurdles on their marks around the track. Sandy settled into her start lane position, nervous but intent. "Well, let's see," I told Coach M. and then walked across the infield so I could film her hurdle form down the backstretch. With the gun, four racers charged at spaced intervals around the first turn. By the time they passed me, Sandy and Carrie had already built a lead on their competitors, with Sandy a few strides faster than her more experienced teammate. She charged the hurdles, as was her nature, drove the lead leg up before the barrier and set sail, arcing over with way too much clearance and arms flying out to the sides. Coming down with a backward lean and landing a flat foot in front of her center of mass, she wobbled, gathered and launched toward the next hurdle. She circled the track this way, sprinting, then sailing, sprinting, then sailing again. Despite the awkward form, the others steadily faded behind her. In unadorned fashion, she won, bent over afterward with a sheepish grin and a time just two tenths of a second shy of the Sectional Championship standard.

Toward meet's end, on the far side of the track, Tammi shook her arms a few times and took a step back from the start line of the 3000m. Alongside was a teammate but no others. Henninger had entered no one in the event. This was Tammi's only competitive effort of the day, and we were hoping the opportunity to run it fresh in perfect conditions, with no competitive pressure and an assured victory, would allow her to simply enjoy an effort that contained the best kinds of motion. That was the hope.

Her first laps went well. She came through the 1600m mark on pace for a solid personal time, one far faster than her Indoor Track's best effort. Each time around, I hollered encouragements, but in the hard laps that followed she began slowing. The arms lowered, the legs cycled more slowly through their strides, and her eyes projected worry. Teammates on the other side of the track cheered her on, but still the lap seconds swelled. She passed me one last time, fight-less, and I called out again. Though she won, there was no surge around the final turn, no strong push across the finish line, just a suffered pace until the distance finally ran out. Distracted with gathering the 4x400 relay on the track for their final event, I turned to find her nowhere nearby. Coach Mercado, though, had heard her mutter as she walked off, "I'm done."

The official fired the gun, and I followed our opening leg of the relay around the first turn and down the backstretch. Then I saw her standing out there, alone, aside the far turn of the track. Her hands hung limply at her side, and her head was bowed. She resembled someone in prayer—or maybe just someone contemplating a warm spring day.

Terry

The hot May sun had punched up afternoon temperatures as the girls tallied their 200-meter workout intervals. They were completing only a few, but for the work to work, all had to be at a specified pace. Halfway through their sweaty labors, they suddenly were not hitting that pace.

I had seen this before, how an unspoken consensus can permeate a group, and the group simple decides, without vote or acclamation, to dampen things down, to hold back. But they had been warned about the consequence of failure. As the lead group shuffled off from a decidedly lackluster interval, I double-checked the watch. "That's too slow," I shouted after them. "It doesn't count." There was a short pause, then someone's voice reverberated back across the infield a little too loudly. "F—k you." A few minutes later, I had told Terry to take the rest of the day off, as many days off, in fact, as needed to polish her grammatical skills and return to me with a written apology.

After practice, Coach Delsole was walking with me out to the parking lot. He'd watched the whole affair and could barely contain his amusement. "Yeah, well I'm glad you enjoyed it," I replied to his smirk. As I bent to open my car trunk, Coach called out quietly from his truck nearby. "Hey coach?"

"What?" I answered briskly, still annoyed.

"F—k you."

I didn't turn around, but I could hear him chuckling.

Terry had always been righteously adamant about things. And early in her high school running career, on one point she was emphatically clear. She was going to be a long sprinter. There was a lot of basic speed there, but I knew, given her size and genetic background, she would not become the highly competitive 200/400 track racer she saw as her future. Terry, though, didn't agree and scoffed at the notion of extending her range to the 800-meter event. But I insisted, so during her freshman and sophomore years, she begrudgingly clocked the occasional pedestrian times at that distance. The fact she made the state championship in the 400 meter her sophomore year seemed to bolster her case, but by then Coach D. and I had already pulled an end-around. During the indoor track season earlier that year, we had nudged her up to the 600-meter event, where she made the state championship. Her junior year, she went states again in the 600m, and then she popped a significant 800m in winning a spring Outdoor Track invitational. Even those successes, though, failed to tilt the argument for the 800 at the Open Qualifier meet that June. Insistent, she finished third in the 400 meter qualifier event and sat home during states.

Her senior year of Indoor Track, Terry 'went states' again in the 600m, but this time added the 300m as well. She could have insisted *I told you so* and judged the argument over. It wasn't. Runners take their own time, so Coach and I continued the progression. Terry ran her 200's and 400's, but she put in a leg of the 4x1500m event at the early-season CNS Relays. Short on sprinters, she took up duties on the 4x100 relay. At the Chittenango Invitational, she won the 400m, but a few days later, she doubled in the 1500/800m events against a league competitor, winning both. On it went, the mix of events. When the league championship rolled around, she placed only third in the 400m. For the Sectional Championship, I told her she was needed in the 800m, and she placed third with a school record time six seconds faster than her previous PR, an effort worth six team points. Ten days later at the State Qualifier Meet, she'd made a decision, and that led to another school record in the 800m and no one in front of her when she crossed the finish line. Terry headed to states, and in that talented New York field, she finished 11th, her best state championship performance in five trips. Four college years later, Terry raced the D3 national championship 800m. I saw her a few years after her college graduation. By then, she was well into a career in accounting. She didn't mind the long hours, the hard work needed to master her profession.

"But," she admitted, "I'd like to be racing again."

***

Sandy had a track-related problem that demanded some time and talk, so once everyone but the modified girls running intervals had left the track, the two of us leaned against the stadium stands and weighed the pros and cons of her competitive choices in the championships ahead. The day has slipped a notch from the outright gorgeousness of our Wednesday league meet day—clouds reoccupied the place-- but this was still a dandy, with mild enough temperatures and scant winds. Tomorrow's similar forecast suggested that a string of bona fide spring days was probable.

Sandy's debut in the 400-meter intermediate hurdles at our final league meet was everything I expected it to be—and more. Coach Delsole had been right, but her successful introduction to the event came with a problem. In the coming league championship, her favored 400 meter event was immediately before the 400 hurdles. That close together, she couldn't do both. She had to choose.

I had already taken the long view. "Honest truth," I told her first-hand, "you're not a raw speed person, a 100m or 200m racer. You are more of a long-sprinter, and college coaches, if you run in college, will see you that way and even move you up in distance as you develop more power and strength-endurance." Sandy didn't disagree. I discussed her slowly improving 400m times and what that might portend for her current competitiveness if the open 400m remained her focus as a senior the following year. Sandy listened and nodded.

The modified kids pattered to their finishes and assembled in a large circle on the infield for drills. I told Sandy that nothing was a given, that the 400 hurdles was simply one of those tough events that quickly spit out pretenders. She already knew that anything one time around the track full bore, whether with hurdles or not, was going to be hard. If she chose the 400 hurdles, I said, she would be joining more distance speed-based workouts her senior year to increase her overall power. Sandy gave that some thought, then she told me, "Coach Mercado's sprint workouts are good, but I just don't have to work as hard in them." Remembering her on all fours after several of the distance interval practices she joined--and knowing that she did not measure herself as your typical runner does—on the question of the 400 hurdles, I took that as yes.

***

If you glanced at the on-line results of our Friday night Arcaro Invitational, you saw everything that someone thought you wanted to know—meet results. But you actually would have missed a lot. For instance, you could easily fail to notice that, of all our event entries, not a single one was a senior. None. Noting that, you might have been curious enough to consult our school calendar and discover that this Friday was also the date of the Senior Ball. And as Coach D. or I could have told you, the Ball is simply one of those special moments in a student-athlete's life to which we automatically concede. There are others.

None of our athletes scored higher than 5th overall in their events, which might also prompt someone to conclude the meet was less than a stellar effort for our team. That, though, would also be a mistake. With our seniors dancing it up elsewhere, Coach M. and I had the opportunity to learn a little more about our young understudies. If asked, we could have explained all the bright spots and signs of emerging talent and aptitude we watched from the infield. We were, in effect, getting a peak at the future, a future never assured, but at least possible.

Chrissy, our aspiring freshman pole vaulter, had persevered through the growing pains of learning a highly technical event that also demanded adept athletic skills. Fickle upstate weather seldom helps in that difficult training. Some days, when the rain flies, even making the meet's opening height is a feat for the neophytes, so Chrissy's half-foot improvement, her next important notch up, suggested we might just have a vaulter for the future. And when Lori clocked a personal record in the 800m, it seemed as though the middle-distance hook had been set. She was progressing from the *can-I-do-it* stage to a *yes-I-can* one. All she needed was to remain faithful to her potential.

Coach Corley, meanwhile, had placed our 8th grader, Peter, in the 1600m, where he would toe the line with a field full of veteran racers. It was time. We had always counselled those selectively classified 8th graders and their parents that the highest priority for young athletes was to first learn how to train on the varsity level. Successful competing came second. Peter had handled the training well and had also notched some solid competitive efforts in his first varsity season. Obviously aware of his gifted aerobic ability, I had been quietly tutoring him on that persistent misconception of distance runners as simply robust aerobic machines. Success also requires basic foot-speed, the ability to cycle through strides quickly and efficiently. "You're going to get tired of hearing me talk about developing more basic speed," I had warned Peter earlier in the season. But he was unfazed, ready for the challenge.

By the time the field circled into their second lap under the stadium, the hard chargers were rhythmically clicking off the meters even as they jockeyed for positions and waited to make their moves. Behind those front runners followed a cadre of chasers, racers with no illusions of top positions, just besting the clock and their closest competitors. And toward the back came Peter. He was straining for all he was worth, bound for no ribbon or break-out performance or even a seasonal PR. Still, he charged on, immersed in the task of minutes and seconds and becoming a better racer. The field circled into their bell lap. Peter, far off the leaders, dug down in his final back-straight, reaching for that foot-speed he'd been promised was coming.

[175]

***

A steady rain fell all morning. That afternoon, arriving at the high school for our Monday practice, the rain had intensified to a downpour. For a few moments before going inside, I stood on the track, water pounding on my parka hood, and I wondered what could be usefully accomplished in that monsoon to prepare for Thursday's league championship. The answer was nothing, so I moved the interval workout inside.

Following attendance and warm-ups, our shrunken championship distance squad sat in the alcove hallway aside Cafeteria II. That was our indoor home for bad-weather workouts on The Oval, a familiar hallway circuit. No one had lobbied for heading out into the rain with its thirty mile an hour wind gusts. Stuffy halls and T-shirts were considered preferable.

The month before, almost to the day, they had completed a similar workout out on the track. Only a few variables had changed. The obvious variable, I told them, was fitness. They were in better shape and would be stronger. Secondly, on the track that day, they had run their three sets with a longer recovery between the 800 and 400 meter efforts in each set than they would get in our hallways. That would amplify fatigue and dampen times. Then there was the matter of turns, where the gradual arches of the outdoor track were replaced by the hard 90° hallway corners. Those needed to be 'softened' by running the apex and reducing the tangential forces pushing them outward, also slowing times. Most of the indoor track veterans had mastered apex running, but the technique only helped so much. The faster the speed, the more difficult those corners would become. So, their four-lap 800m times would suffer less for hall running than their quicker 400's. They knew that too.

The troops gathered into their groups and positioned themselves at the start, instinctively lining up faster to slower. They needed no prodding. The shifting of particular runners from group to group—those earlier experiments to test and to encourage—were over. These were, after all, the championship squads.

As the wind-driven rain hammered against the windows, they set off on their first 800m effort. Matt launched himself first. Luke, Aidan, Peter and Jack opened strong but were in Matt's rearview mirror by the end of lap three. Peter was also quickly left behind, but what might have appeared to be merely an off day for him was more likely a first-timer's encounter with basic physiology. We had seen it often enough with others to understand. Younger runners, despite any amount of talent, simply have not acquired a reward afforded the veterans, the accumulation of miles and seasons--and the maturity that creates power. If Renato Canova is right, if every event is an event of extension where training allows one to hold a desired race incrementally longer, then so too is the effect of seasons and miles. The more of both you gain over the years and seasons, the more the body adjusts to the load, and the less the accumulations produce lingering fatigue. Peter, nearing the end of his first varsity season, was simply getting tired. Watching him circle, working hard, I knew we needed to carefully monitor his rest and recovery--and I wondered what this meant for the championships ahead.

Lori ran as though she should mimic Matt's position for the girls, surging her way ahead of a chase group which included Tammi, Pam, Cindy and Erin. In the first 800, she finished three seconds ahead of her teammates—and twenty-three seconds faster than her first 800 in that April workout. I thought that might set the tone for the afternoon, but her teammates reeled her in on the 400 interval, all finishing in a tight clump that sent another message. While the boys' front runners gradually strung out through the subsequent sets, the girls gave each other no quarter, jostling turns in tight formations, jockeying for positions down the straights, creating their own monsoon of motion. Between sets, hands on knees, they made eye contact with each other and nodded wordlessly. By the end, the too-tight 400m efforts were, as expected, about the same as the earlier April workout, but their 800's averaged twelve seconds faster. Almost every runner who completed both workouts had improved dramatically. With interval times logged on my workout sheet and satisfied with themselves, the girls jogged a relaxed, chatty cool-down together. It had been a performance as admirable, in its own way, as a school record, an effort worth watching. Wendy, though, was still somewhere far away.

***

With two days of easier work to recover, the runners arrived rested and ready for their league championship. The afternoon before I had told them, "The hay is in the barn," then noted the squinted, perplexed eyes and so explained the old adage. By the time our teams unloaded at the Liverpool High School site, amiable afternoon temperatures in the mid-sixties had begun a slow decline. The winds, though, were diminished, and no rain threatened, so an opportunistic race day was in the offing. This championship had no event standards. Coaches had the freedom to enter any two athletes in each individual event, so we continued our practice of balancing a total team effort with the chance to give some hardworking individuals their first-- or only--championship opportunity. For some, it meant a last shot at achieving the required standards for the Section III Class AA or Open Qualifier meets coming up. Both team buses had brimmed with hopes and expectations.

On time, Lori settled into the blocks for the 100 high hurdles of the pentathlon, the meet's first event. Earlier in the season, Lori had decided that was her event, and she made her intentions clear. Maybe she had watched Katie adopt the pentathlon the previous year and finish 5th at leagues, with teammates cheering her on under the lights as she gutted out the finish of the 800 meter, the final of five events and a long competitive day. Maybe Lori liked what she saw about the overall toughness of those athletes and wanted a piece of it. Regardless, all season we carried on a respectful disagreement about her short and long-term prospects in the event. But I had finally capitulated, and so with time found to practice the basics of the five events, there she was at last, springing from the blocks at the gun and muscling her way over ten hurdles to place fourth and tally the points earned for her modest time. In the pentathlon, athletes gain performance points for each of the five events, so while you compete against others, what really matters at the end of the day is the point total. Lori pulled on her sweats, gave me that not-great-but-not-too-bad look and walked off to get water. She still had the high jump, shot put, long jump and 800 meter. She was just getting started.

The early events for the combined girls/boys meet were, like Lauren's hurdles, neither disappointing nor spectacular. The athletes performed well enough, with some scoring top-6 finish points for their teams and others pushing hard but coming in lower. Coach Corley had both Matt and Peter in the 1600 meter, and they shook out with strides on the infield before reporting to the official at the start. Matt had surveyed the field, knew his chances and thought through his tactics. In previous season's that would have meant going hard in the early laps—right off the leaders or maybe even leading—and then hanging on. More often than not, the strategy meant struggling the last lap while others passed him, a tactic coaches seldom advise unless they know something the athlete doesn't. After a few seasons of such disappointments, though, Matt had made some decisions. He had pushed his weak spots in practices, accomplishing what is called 'finding the race in the workout.' He had tacked extra miles on to some general conditioning runs. And he had learned how to bear down. He was trying, in effect, to transform a weakness into a strength, and he was making progress.

The field jostled its way around the first lap, and Matt slipped into a comfortable spot up among the leaders. In the second lap, the sorting began in earnest, with some runners falling off, others pushing up into strategic positions. Everyone waited. Peter maneuvered in the middle, resisting the temptation to push too hard too early, reminding himself to stay relaxed, to show patience. Matt maneuvered himself near the front chargers, rhythmically smooth and bidding his time. They circled. Near the end of lap three, the game finally unfolded as fatigue and talent separated pretenders from contenders. Matt already knew who the players would be, and he guarded his position with the front-runners. It was a small group by then, three or four. As they passed into the bell lap, I clicked the third lap time on my stopwatch but didn't bother looking. Only the race mattered. Out of the first curve and into the final back stretch, the old Matt would have slowed and strained. We would have watched competitors bully by him in the final three hundred meters. But this was a different day and a different Matt. Down the backstretch, a strong F-M lead racer gapped the front group, leaving Matt and the rest battling for second. They hit the 200-meter mark, the psychological go-point. Matt dug down around the final turn, edging ahead of the three others. They came around and barreled down the final straight, arms and legs pumping furiously. In the finish sprint, Matt was not losing meters to his rivals; he was opening on them. He crossed in second with a personal record, a top-5 sectional time, and a weary smile. Peter soon zoomed across, arms now flapping tiredly at his side. The more experienced field had swallowed him. He placed only 9th, but with the fastest 8th grade time in the section.

Just past the midway point of the meet, with Lori already placing third in both the high jump and shot put pentathlon events, I stood on the infield with Cindy. I was explaining how capable she was, how well she would perform if she put herself in the game with a strong first four hundred meters. The wide-eyed look I received back was the same offered before in the cold months of indoor track, just before she had stepped out to tackle her first 3000m. But now, that wide-eyed response seemed more confident. She had proved as much at the ESM Invitational two weeks earlier, pushing the third 200m of her eight hundred meter race, taking a chance in the hardest part and, despite fading down the homestretch, fighting her way to a personal record and the Sectionals qualifying standard. Five days after that, she had set another personal record in the 1500m, where she had even led teammate Lori until being chased down in the final 300 meters. And then again, with yet another personal record in the 800m at the cold and breezy Arcaro Invitational. The cautious Lori of Indoor Track seemed gone, replaced by someone unafraid to put herself into pain's way, someone willing to override the internal warning signals of mid-race, taking the chance by trusting the training. She wasn't close to the section's fastest 800m runners, but she was poised with the right attitude.

When the gun went off, the runners whisked around turn one, and I was not surprised to see Cindy clamped on to the back of the front pack, which had already been gaped by the streaking F-M race favorite. They circled around, with Cindy swelling the chase pack, on pace for a personal record. Out of turn one and into the backstretch, she swung out and passed a runner. Down the backstretch, she pushed hard and passed another. And then another. Suddenly, she was threatening to take over 2nd, with the F-M front-runner already six seconds gone, way out in front. Into the final turn, though, Cindy began struggling. Her form broke down slightly; the stride lengthened, and her turn-over rate decreased. One girl re-passed her, then another. But she was still driving until, inexplicably, only fifteen meters from the finish, she simply crashed down forward, as though desire had outrun gravity. She hit the track's infield curb. Stunned, she rolled over. "Get up!" I screamed from nearby, and she rose, dazed. "Finish!" I yelled, and she stumbled her way across the line, still managing a top-six finish.

I rushed to her side and noted only minor leg abrasions--no blood. "Are you O.K.?" I asked. She nodded she was all right. A competitor came over and bent above her. "Oh, I'm sorry; that was so bad," she told Cindy, patting her on the back. I thought about the risks taken, the gamble that almost paid off. "No," I insisted, "that was great!" Her competitor starred at me curiously.

Toward meet's end, Wendy lined up with others on the far side of the track for the 3000m. She had returned from her family trip just the day before, so I placed her in that longest event. The time away would have eroded her speed-endurance the most, so the 1500 or 800 meter events were poor options. My choice, though, did not matter. Wendy got out strong and--as usual--raced bravely and with a lot of heart. But by the end she had been lapped by the leaders, finishing almost forty seconds slower than her time a month before on a cold April afternoon. There was no pleasure in my prediction come true. There was nothing to say. I offered her a wordless pat on the shoulder.

It was well into the evening when Lori toed the start line for her final pentathlon event, the 800 meter. The stadium lights were on, and the stands had mostly emptied of spectators. All the pentathlon competitors looked wearied by a long meet of events. Lori forced a slight smile as her teammates shouted encouragement from the infield. She had not done well in the high jump event and needed a strong effort on this run for the points that could push her up in the final standings. When the official fired them off, the small, intrepid group of competitors surged around the first turn, casting long shadows under the lights. Lori paced confidently near the front. When they strode around for the bell lap, one circuit left to their five-event day, she pushed into the lead, surged along the back stretch and never looked back. Teammates whooped her down the front straight for a five second win, enough points, in the final tally, to push her into third place. She stood off the track on the infield, smiling and accepting congratulations under the stadium lights--just as she might have imagined.

***

The hard part is telling certain athletes they were good enough for one championship but not the next. The required Sectional Championship event standards, of course, always make that point all by themselves, with no empathy or pity. There is no way, after all, an athlete is going to argue with numbers on a printed page. You can't plead your case with a stopwatch or a tape measure. All season, Coach M. and I had made efforts to provide athletes the opportunities to reach those sectional standards. In a few instances, we had warned athletes of the urgency to train strategically and compete with maximum efforts if they wanted to be on that sectionals team bus. Some came close, just not close enough. In the end, the clock and the tape measure decided who was on the bus and who wasn't.

By mid-afternoon of our practice time the day after leagues, the sky cleaved to open blue and temperatures climbed to the low sixties. But there were strong wind gusts, as though clearing things out for what lay ahead. Ten athletes had handed in their uniforms. The team shrank to fifteen--fewer still.

For the sectional championship, I had asked the athletes to develop event plans, something more specific than trying hard and hoping good things happen. A race plan, we know, can focus the mind, calm the athlete, and often, by looking back afterword, reveal the path forward. Race plans are another form of mental mapping and are integral to sustained competitive success. But because goals also establish accountability, some of the less experienced or less invested runners resist them. They don't want results to answer for, except privately. Since make-a-wish racing seldom works in the long run, by sectionals most of those plan-less runners are no longer climbing onto the team bus.

Good years or bad, I have always told the athletes, the sectional championship is the one we hang our hat on, the time when a total team effort matters most. That means creating the strongest event roster possible—the coaches' jobs—and the athletes doing all they can to maximize the team effort. Personal desires or goals matter less than team points. Sometimes, in this day and age, that's a hard sell for youngsters who have been feed a steady diet of individualism--and the situation is not helped by others who insist that track and field is an "individual sport." So sometimes there are unhappy faces when an athlete is told he or she won't run their favorite event. That's when I have to remind them privately that this is the sectional championship.

Other times, though, individual and team needs align nicely. The events the athletes want to contest well are exactly the events where we need them. We needed Pam this day to perform her best in the 1500m and, with a full effort, score team points. Pam wanted a qualifying standard for the Open Qualifier meet she had never reached. Pam had even emailed a plan the morning of the meet:

For my 1500 today I would like to try to be around 5:03. My splits last week were right around where I wanted them to be. I think a change I could make is to be at 4:05 on my 3rd lap. Then the last 300m has to be all I have left.

Pam was thinking back to the league championship and her 1500m race there. She had clocked a personal record but finished .16 seconds short of the Open Qualifier standard she wanted. She missed the standard because she paced the first half too fast and then failed to push the third—and mentally hardest—third lap. She had slowed then, hobbled by those internal fears that mounting fatigue likes to foist on distance runners right after mid-race when the end is still too far away. When she did come around to the 1500m start line for her final 300m, she charged ahead with an impressive whirl of arm and leg drive, but by then it was too late. I had told her afterward: even out the lap times, then take the chance in the hard third lap. Push to hold pace there, and you will hit the standard. She did not have much say about that strategy, but I sensed the advice had made an impression.

The day we always imagined for a sectional championship was warm, sunny and windless. We got two of three. After deboarding from the team bus, Coach M. and I seated them in the stands where shade extended from the looming press boxes above. By the meet's 4:30 p.m. start, cloud cover made that as unnecessary as my earlier speech about not baking in the sun. And in the comfortable high 60's weather, the stadium flags hung limp.

By the time Pam stepped from the infield to the 1500m start line, the team had already scored points, not many, but at least a few in each of the preceding three events. Riley's 100 high hurdles had provided the most excitement. The year before, she had not even

[186]

qualified for the event. This season, with form and speed honed by diligent practice, she powered her hurdles and placed top-6 with a personal record while meeting the standard for the Open Qualifier meet. Her trifecta prompted a smile wider than the track.

The official called the 1500m field to the start line. Six of them had raced for their Fayetteville-Manlius and Liverpool teams in the cross-country national championship the previous December. The event was packed with talent, and Pam stood nervously behind that curved start-line of strong racers. We made brief eye contact, and I merely nodded.

With the official's command, the racers stepped forward, crouched at the start-line, then leapt off with the gun's sharp discharge. Pam jostled with others for position down the backstretch, then settled in behind the leaders group. First laps are often just about staying out of trouble, avoiding being boxed in or clipped by another runner's strides while trying to set the proper pace. Pam found a safe position, and as she circled around into lap two, I stood down-track fifteen meters from the start line and barked out her lap time. She was a second and a half slower than her fast first lap at leagues--perfect.

Second lap, the runners parceled out their energy stores and assumed or searched positions for the hard laps ahead. Pam came through a half second faster than her league's 800 meter mark. Where she had slowed by almost seven seconds on her league's second lap, this time it was two. She was dictating her race rather than merely responding. It was a fast field, and clearly only a heroic effort would win her a top-6 finish. I waited as she headed into the tough third lap. Let's see, I thought to myself, let's see. The front runners bore down, shaking off a few pretenders. Pam hung with those and came through the third lap a second and a half under the target time she had emailed me that morning. "Go!" was all I yelled, knowing she'd taken the risk and pushed back on the fear. The rest would just be heart and guts. The lead runners were already fighting each other down the front straight as Pam drove through the final curve. Her form remained strong and efficient. Summoning up all her reserves, she chased runners down the straight, crossing the line out of the top six but with a time that would send her to the Open Qualifier. I stopped for a moment on the infield to jot down split times. Pam stood bent over on the track, gulping air. Then she straightened and, with a tired tilt, walked toward me. Even from a distance, I saw the weary smile.

The meet moved on and proved that we simply lacked the talent to compete across multiple events with the stronger and deeper teams. Some of the athletes failed, for one reason or another, to bring out their best when it mattered most. The top-5 team finish I thought possible eluded us. Coach and I had to watch Wendy struggle to last place in the 1500m, almost seventeen seconds slower than her seasonal best. The end we feared had come. Still, two of the team's relays and another individual clocked seasonal best performances and punched their tickets to the Open Qualifier. Then, late in the meet, after the lights came on, Lori again stood on the line with other tired pentathlon competitors, waiting on the gun for their final 800 meter event. In a tougher field this week, Lori would drop two notches in the final results and fail to achieve the point total standard needed for that next step to Open Qualifiers. Her pentathlon experiment for the season would be over. But she would score team points, and she would always be able to recall that last view around her final turn as she bore down on a finish line under stadium lights with no one in front of her.

Coach Delsole

After each event heat of our dual meets, the finish line is typically a confusion of timers trying to get finish places and times correct while surrounded by tired but curious athletes. We had decided for the non-scoring, JV-level heats to time by lanes rather than places. It sped up the process, and so the meet. Coach Delsole had his lane assignment, and he also verified the finish orders if necessary. He has a good eye for that.

Robbie had been with the team a couple of seasons. He had some learning challenges but was a good kid and a hard worker. The sport was a great opportunity for him. Robbie, though, could be impatient or even insistent. So, when he crossed the line after a solid effort, tired as he was, he immediately wanted to know his time. We typically shoe the runners away as the timers huddle to make sure everything is correctly recorded on the meet sheet. I was recording the times and names offered by the timers. Robbie kept hovering and insisting. Coach was standing close by, waiting his turn. He gave a fake, studied glance at his watch. "Robbie," he announced, "that was your fastest time of the year." Ecstatic, Robbie twirled, all smiles, and, as we finished up undistracted, he pranced off toward the infield.

When we were ready for the next heat, I turned to Coach. "You had no idea what his time was, did you?"

Coach had been watching Robbie jog happily away. He glanced again at his stopwatch, where nothing stared back but rows of zeros. "Nope," he said, with a wry smile.

***

Parents:
With yesterday's sectional championship, we have completed
our team season. It was a good one, characterized by the strong
practice efforts, enthusiasm and improving event performances by
the athletes. Coach Mercado and I appreciated how the girls battled
early-season weather fluctuations and then a steady diet of rain to
achieve their best dual-meet record in the past three years. Most of
the athletes set personal records in one or more events, and we had
a large number adopting new events that contributed to competitive
efforts. I reviewed our team records from the past decade. This
season, we had the lowest percentage of students dropping from
the team in those first weeks, a signal of the perseverance and
investment of this group. While we'll miss our graduates, this is a
team destined to return stronger and more competitive in 2020 and
beyond.

Thanks for the support. I hope you enjoyed the season also.

Coach Vermeulen

***

Coach for enough scholastic seasons, and you eventually discard most pretentions about your ultimate powers of persuasion. Personalities and attitudes show up at afternoon practices that are, despite the popular mythologies, close to fully formed. Even on the scholastic level, we illuminate the characters of athletes more than we create them. So, if we pay attention, it should not be surprising when the athletes ultimately decide what levels of practice effort and competitive accomplishment matters to them. Some coaches specifically recruit those highly committed team members and then pretend authorship.

There are multiple finish lines to most scholastic track and field seasons, various ways to declare victory. For some athletes, making the league or sectional championship represents a personal pinnacle of success. That's enough for the season, they declare one way or another—and in achieving that goal, they deserve a tip of the hat similar to those for which it's the state championship or failure. The teammates who surround the athlete can certainly affect his or her decisions about goals. Sports are, after all, communal. The projected standards and expectations of coaches can likewise expand or dampen the athlete's enthusiasm for developing full potential. Ultimately, though, it's the inner desire to achieve individually or with teammates on a relay that directs the vision and the efforts of the distance runner. No one puts in the hours to clock a superlative race effort on the track just as a favor or to fulfill someone else's expectation. Competitive effort needs to be in the blood, a form of self-definition.

The Open Qualifier meet of late May or early June, our New York gateway to the State Championship, sings its unique tune. The team season is over. The fraction of section's team athletes moving on to the Open Qualifier meet may be ten percent at best. It could just as easily be five. The stadium stands sit half full even as the stakes rise for fewer athletes. The athletes responding to that siren call of personal greatness have arrived by different paths and for different reasons. Some have worked seasons and years just for an outside shot at making the state championship. In exotic territory, this is their moment. Others have already been there in previous years, gone home disappointed, and returned with more training and hardened resolve. For others still, the elite few, the Open Qualifier is almost a foregone conclusion, a steppingstone to loftier goals on the state and national championship stages. And there are always those that coaches describe as "just happy to be there," athletes with no expectations beyond arriving at that stadium on that singular day in a school singlet to toe the start line. All of the competitors, though, have made their decisions and all have made sacrifices.

Twelve of our girls team members arrived at Cicero-North Syracuse's Richard Nastasi Stadium to compete in three relays and seven individual events. None were favored to win and advance, but all had earned their shot. They were joined by several on the boys team. It was a mellow day, an afternoon that prompts thoughts of the long, lazed summer weeks ahead. Temperatures hovered in the mid to high sixties, and light breezes nudged scattered clouds. The stadium, a week removed from boisterous sectional championship spectators and screaming teammates, adopted a more workmanlike demeanor as the process of sorting out the best was set to proceed. Each division, large schools and small, would advance one athlete per event to the state championship. A third could qualify if they met their division's event standard and were the next highest division finisher. And this year, super-qualifiers could be added if he or she had posted an extraordinary performance sometime in the season at a large invitational.

Coach and I had preached. We had presented the visions, the possibilities, the strategies. Over the years, I had watched dreams both realized and dreams dashed at this strange outcast of a competition just beyond the 'team season.' One thing was always clear when the gun sounded for the first event. All the mental and physical momentum from that point on belonged to the athletes. Coaches could offer reminders, tactical advice and last-minute encouragement, but beyond that they were relegated to cheerleading.

With the national anthem rendered, the meet began. Our 4x800, 4x100 and 4x400 meter relays all gave good efforts, but none raced their fastest and all raced out of the money. Our two hundred-meter sprinters both qualified for finals but both finished deep in the pack, with no trip to states. The same proved true for Jackie in the 400 meter. Event by event, seasons ended.

Pam and Matt were competing in their respective 1500m and 1600m races. Even with similar training, they had nevertheless arrived through different circumstances. Matt, up first, had seen his streak of strong finishes diminished the week before by a sectional championship 1600m effort a few seconds slower than his best. That led to a disappointing 5th place finish. Just a glitch we had wondered? A bad night's sleep or something as apparently innocuous as a momentary lapse of attention in some part of a lap that became consequential? I was not sure, and Matt offered no analysis. Over the season, though, he had accomplished something that might easily go unnoticed if time and place were the only measures. His M.O. the previous seasons, despite stated intentions to the contrary, had been to push hard early in races only to flag in the final meters, to overestimate his reserves or resistance to pain. Typically, the view of his final turns before the finish straight had been of racers pulling by him. There would be solemn, perplexed expressions afterward.

That had changed this season, though in undramatic fashion. We didn't talk about it much, but Matt had begun hanging on longer in races—and then beating some challengers to the line. He even reversed roles sometimes, becoming the stalker, overtaking others in the final meters. It was a shift as attitudinal as it was physical. He had managed, through his own decisions and efforts, to turn that racing liability into a strength. And because many racers in those circumstances merely settle and rationalize them, the change was something to be admired.

Strengths, though, have to be permanent, and they need to be predictable. That is evident with those we like to call "money racers," and I was hoping Matt would be showing money in a critical race. Coming around the first turn after the gun, he held a safe position. Through the first lap, and then the second, he was in the thick of the race, chasing the leaders not far ahead. But in the third lap, something changed. He backed off the pace and slowed, like a Formula 1 car which had miscalculated fuel in the final circuit and was sputtering. The leaders opened daylight on him, which in the final lap became a significant gap. Through the last turn, he got passed. He crossed the line well behind and was again silent and perplexed. He'd lost something more important than a race, and now had a long summer ahead to think about what that was.

Most of us like to believe in the "ah-hah moment." That supposed transformational experience when everything suddenly changes for the better is intoxicatingly attractive because it eliminates the responsibility of time. Somebody is something one moment, then, through a magical physical or mental experience, instantly becomes something better. We like to believe in that possibility, and we often pretend it actually occurs. Ah-hah moments, however, do not exist for distance runners. Revelatory thoughts seldom precipitate inspirational actions. It's actually the opposite. Out of prolonged work completed repetitiously over time come the notions of champions, not vice versa. Distance athletes facing their running futures do not suddenly create; they slowly discover. Sometimes, coaches hardly figure into that process.

When the gun sounded for Pam a short time later, I wondered if her successful gambit of the week before had taught that hers was not really a gamble, just a possible sacrifice she had the capacity to recreate. I was hoping one discovery would lead to others. But she went out too fast again, then ballooned her times in the middle laps, as though afraid again, before powering home in the final meters when it was too late, slower than just the week before. She never came close to her best possible effort. She raced as though another gambit was not worth the doubt, as though once had been enough. Afterward, she gathered her sweats and had little to say. Her season was over.

And so, with Peter still training for the National Middle School Mile two weeks away, we were down to a team of one.

Most of the afternoon, Aggie Stadium in Greensboro, North Carolina had rocked with a swollen national championship crowd, a DJ blasting tunes beneath the stands and constant action on the track. But by the time Peter arrived with his parents at four o'clock for the Middle School National Mile, many of the marquee events had been contested and the stands had begun emptying. His 5:50 event was delayed, so we had extra time. I walked him around, showing him the bathrooms, the warm-up and clerking area, and a place to relax out of the sun under the stands.

At 5:00 p.m., I sent him out to loosen up and prepare. After, we reported to the clerking area just as the girls' freshman mile began two events ahead of his, only to discover they'd already clerked the boys Middle School mile group. The lady at the desk, though, merely checked him off and told him to hang around as the racers would soon be queued. Nervous, but excited, Peter completed striders in the grass behind the stadium until his event was called a few minutes later. I watched as the racers were seated in rows of chairs under a small tent and then individually called up to receive their bib numbers.

"One on each hip and one above the heart," the official directed the young competitors once all had received their numbers. "If you don't know where your heart is, I'll help you find one." Peter smiled and stuck on his numbers. I edged up, patted him good luck on the shoulder and left to take a spot in the stadium stands along the backstretch of the track.

Soon enough, his heat was led out, then slow-walked down the back stretch and around the first curve to a final queue. Up in the stands, his parents and a few relatives shouted and waved. By the time Peter stepped to the start-line after seven, the sun was lowering, and the stadium with its sparse crowd had assumed a comparative evening calm. Shadows from the press-box above stretched all the way across the infield to the backstretch where I stood.

Peter got out well, but by the 200-meter mark he had been swallowed by a pack chasing the leaders. He had nowhere to move, no daylight either in front or beside him, just a mass of cycling legs and arms hemming him in. For the first 800 meters, he remained stuck, only breaking out in the middle of lap three. By then, his lap times had ballooned, and the leaders had paced away in front of him. He surged with everything left, his last lap five seconds faster than his third, but he proved again that catch-up in the middle-distance races is never an effective race strategy.

As he trudged off the evening infield, I motioned him to side steps into the stands. For a few moments, we sat alone and chatted. "First of all," I told him, "congratulations on a great season." I asked what he thought of the race, and he offered a chagrined remark about being boxed in. He knew. "I felt comfortable, but I couldn't move."

I merely nodded. "Yes, you lost time in those laps. And in a championship race, you never want to be too comfortable; you want to be competitive. In championships, you sometimes need to take risks."

He sat and mulled. The sun had lowered and the lengthening shadows engulfed the stands. So far from home, so far from the snows of early March. "When you come back down next year, you'll race that way," I promised him. "It only gets better."

Then I sent him to his parents, waiting with their hugs and their congratulations.

Kerry

Attempt #1 at Outdoor Nationals ended in water. A torrid of rainwater. Someone squeezed the celestial sponges again and again as the low-lying stadium track began to fill and events were halted. Puddles swelled, linked, deepened. I noted the irony as flooding advanced to the edge of the steeplechase water pit, paused, then spilled in. Within an hour, darkness had descended, and the stadium below became a shallow lake, populated only by a few splashing athletes instead of ducks. The meet events, including Kerry's steeplechase competition, were postponed until the next morning. Regents exams, however, prohibited a rescheduled flight, so her running year went under with everything else.

Kerry tried again as a senior. It wasn't easy getting back. Her promising Fall cross-country season succumbed to illness at Sectionals, as she failed in her final attempt to make a State Championship. Ten days before the Indoor Track State Qualifier, she was diagnosed with a stress fracture and stood on the sidelines several weeks into the outdoor season. Spring went hard. Behind in training, she plugged on, slowly earning back lost fitness.

The weather warmed. As she worked, some teammates surrendered to senioritis, accepted lackluster seasons, and handed in uniforms. Kerry mustered resolve and pushed harder. She qualified a second time for nationals, then trained alone for two weeks. In mid-June, seven days before graduation, she returned to North Carolina. The lake had drained. Saturday evening, a soft southern breeze meandered through the stadium, and when the gun for her seeded heat cracked, the last sunlight of the day had escaped below the tops of trees. Dusk found her circling, fighting the mounting fatigue of land barriers and water jumps, reaching for what was left from a difficult year.

Then it was over. She had a sectional record to take home, and she'd finished seventh in the nation, three tenths of a second from All-American status. I waited by the exit to the infield as she slowly walked away from her final high school competition, utterly spent. As she approached, her head was bowed, but not by regret. When she reached me, she said, "I had no more gears, coach."

Summer

"Life is the sum of all our choices."
—Albert Camus

The roads had already made their choices. Gilly Brook Road decided to marry gravity, quietly weaving fields and sheltering woods in a slow descent. Bennet Corners Road wanted to climb hills instead, skirting lush open meadows and contoured farm fields of energetic corn that, on days when the clouds cooperated, could make your heart ache. On the early mornings when a chill hung in the air, he only had to cinch up a light jacket and make his own choice. There were days, though, with either destination, when he imagined what it might be like to suddenly veer off the shoulder, crossing a meadow of early cows and climbing into the woods beyond, a road mysteriously creating itself before him, and then, once he had passed, dissipating in his wake, like the morning mist lifting.

June

***

One of the problems with our new on-line sports registration program was in the timing. Prospective cross-country runners chatted around tables in the small high school cafeteria, waiting for our early June pre-season meeting to get started, but it would be over a month before the school would activate the on-line system for them to actually sign up. That created the possibility for the new or the less motivated athletes to easily decide our mid-July on-line registration date would be just a dandy time to get serious about distance running. Only it wouldn't be. By that point, a month of critical summer training would have been squandered by the very team members who probably needed it most. So, our early June get-together now had another important purpose besides offering team information. It was also meant to remind everyone that their cross-country season began now, in June.

The showing was small. I scanned for unfamiliar faces, the ones that indicated new athletes who were giving the sport a try. There was always that hope of an unknown ringer, maybe not the annual joke of a "Kenyan transfer student," but the pleasant surprise of an unfamiliar face with potential and something to prove. I recognized all the veterans. I spotted the modified runners I had encouraged, the ones willing to 'move up' to the varsity level. But I saw none of those unfamiliar faces, which meant my letters and emails to several prospects had changed no minds. The architecture of this season's boys and girls teams would be constructed mostly from known parts.

Some of the veterans, though, were missing. One was Sara. A

talented underclassman, she had finished in the team's top-5 the previous season and was poised for greatness. But Coach G. and I had sensed in season that her heart wasn't into distance running. She had signaled that by lagging behind in practice runs that she could have been leading. Her pained look on the trails was common most afternoons. Her mom had promised Coach Gangemi she was working on Sara to give the sport another season, a second shot, but I knew it was a losing battle. The only consolation lay in knowing that her decision was for the best. When a kid requires convincing or coercing to attempt cross-country, trouble looms. A team then inherits a runner who is, at best, tentative, and at worst, someone detrimental to team solidarity. We would at least avoid that. The end result, though, was the girls were down a potential team top-5 runner.

Jackie was also MIA, though her absence less a surprise. Her encouraging sophomore campaign had been followed by a lackluster junior season where Coach G. and I were ineffective in convincing her to push toward her potential. She slogged through submaximal practice efforts and races, and she sank from an expected team top-5 right out of the top-10. The handwriting was on the wall. My attempts to cajole her back for a redemptive third season had likely failed.

And Grace was absent too. Her initial season the year before had started slow, but ended strong, with future potential emanating from her rhythmic and graceful stride. Word would later filter back that she had moved to another district and taken up a different Fall sport. Another what-might-have-been.

Familiar faces, though, were scattered through the small crowd, the faithful who would carry the load, create the teams. One veteran presence, though, was unexpected. Mindy sat passively alone near the side, starring and waiting. The previous year, her dissatisfied mother had led an anti-coach crusade that included a petition full of accusations and misrepresentations that the AD and superintendent judged not credible. A later spring meeting that she demanded with myself and administrators had brought the same result. I met with the AD and superintendent a few days after that meeting to discuss 'better communications,' but we all knew the meeting had been unnecessary and mostly to placate an angry parent. I was convinced we had seen the last of Mindy. She passed on yet another track season where she might have improved basic foot speed. Yet, there she was. *Well*, I thought, *if nothing else, there will be intrigue.*

The girls' circumstances contrasted with the guys. Scattered around tables, they chatted and joked without a care in the world. Their losses to graduation had been minimal, with only one 2018 team top-5 racer headed to college. Like the girls, however, a promising freshman had not returned, lured away by an out-of-season intramural program for another sport, an occurrence increasingly frequent in our district. Despite all the preaching by college coaches, former athletes and sports physiologists about the values of multi-sport participation, our sports teams had become more tribal, not less, because of out-of-season programs. The baseball and lacrosse players that once dotted our program were gone.

The boys, though, were lucky because freshman Peter brought credentials to fill that unexpected void. And with him came another first timer. Long-legged Andy fit the visual prototype of a distance runner, and I hoped the visual was accurate. Another lean and lanky freshman—Trent--sat there also looking the part. Though freshmen are seldom expected to step into scoring roles, we apparently had several with that potential. The closest we were going to come to an unexpected ringer was Peter's brother, who had decided to throw in with the team as a first-season senior. Their senior-freshman brother combination would be odd in that Peter held the upper hand in the running talent department. Ryan, though, was a swimmer at a top sectional level. The mental and physical demands of that sport mirrored running, so we were hoping.

Matt, meanwhile, quietly eyed the crowd, perhaps already plotting a better sports finish than those of his previous indoor and outdoor track seasons. Cross-Country, he freely admitted, was his favorite sport. Redemption was probably part of the seasonal plan. Next to him sat the diminutive and bespeckled Jack, now with a season under his belt, though it had been a tough experience. His 2018 first season had ended prematurely with injury, and I had pointed to his skimpy summer mileage total as the primary cause. Jack had heard enough of that and wasn't looking back. 500 summer miles of preparation had passed under his feet. This season would be different.

The experts on such matters expound on the critical need to create team cultures where members share goals, a mutual work ethic and at least a minimum level of talent. But the reference point for those experts is typically the sports teams that begin their seasons by cutting a percentage of hopefuls who lack that minimum talent level or that proper investment—or both. Those coaches get to shape their rosters initially. Our sport is different. The welcome mat is always out, and no one closes the door with cuts. Inclusive teams such as ours require creating conditions where excellent and average and below average can mutually exist, where a range of talent can succeed together. That's no mean feat, and a glance around the room indicated this would be a season, like many others, of just such a challenge.

I took a breath and called the meeting to order.

All spring during outdoor track, I had offered Cindy reasons to run cross-country in the Fall. The primary argument was that all the mental toughness in the world goes nowhere unless it operates in a body that is physically strong. Cindy needed physical toughness, and I had unabashedly cajoled her all spring about how to develop that. A coach can never know for certain, though, how persuasive such encouragements are with developing runners; they may even have the opposite effect. But I had watched Cindy step to the start line and, fired by inexperience, go at a distance—usually the 800m-- with an admirable boldness. She would charge out with the gun, look for competitors to race and circle that first 400 meters with singular intent. Then, in that infamous third quarter of any race where the mind starts running its calculations and demanding capitulations, Cindy's lack of aerobic fitness would join the internal fear chorus and she'd falter, coming home with a wobble, her head shaking loosely and leaning to one side. Often, neophyte runners initially experimenting with that level of pain quickly join the ranks of overly cautious racers. For just that reason, coaches are supposed to wean such overexuberant foolishness from neophytes. They're supposed to train the proper developmental pacing and use a gradually improving fitness and confidence to bring the times down. That's the way you're supposed to do it.

But I didn't. I just let her go at those 800's. I kept hearing Italian coach Renato Canova declaring, "Every event is an event of extension," and so when Cindy would push hard a little further into subsequent races, I counselled myself patience, time to let fitness catch up to exuberance. Eventually, I hoped, they'd match. The big question was whether she was willing to make the sacrifices and spend the time building the large respiratory engine that would carry her exuberance all the way. Building that aerobic base would require a cross-country season. So all spring I lobbied.

Cindy hemmed and hawed, always good naturedly. She seemed like all the others who think all they need to know is that cross-country is hard. Still, unlike others who shy into other sports because of that thought—or merely shy away--Cindy balanced herself on the fence, slowly performing the subjective calculations to determine if cross-country-hard might, indeed, be in her constitutional wheelhouse. As you could expect from a young adult, she felt her way toward a decision. Rational calculations had little to do with it.

That's what I had hoped, but she was one of the absent faces at our pre-season meeting. She did, though, attend our outdoor track post-season team picnic later that afternoon. Someone must have mentioned the cross-country meeting she'd missed. She was quick to find me and explain that she had been prepping for a final with a teacher. "O.K.," I told her, "Let's have you fill out the cross-country information sheet, so we have contacts for the summer." I fetched the clipboard from the car, gave her both our Basic XC Information and Athlete Information sheets. She returned shortly to hand in the athlete sheet and then, like a proud 5th grader finally trusted with keys to the house, announced, "And I have the other sheet tucked in my pocket so I can't lose it." Then she trotted off to play volleyball with the other girls.

Later, after everyone had eaten and we'd taken our annual picnic Team Photo, I was talking with Coach M. when Cindy came striding toward me, wide-eyed again, intent on something. She waited while Coach and I finished our conversation, and then, not so much as a question, said, "Can we talk about cross-country?"

"Sure," I told her. "We can talk. What's on your mind?"

Cindy paused, collecting her thoughts as though making sure she'd get this right. "Well," she said seriously, "I just want you to know that I don't like running in mud."

***

For two decades, my assistants and I had practiced a June tradition. We called it Packet Night, a mid-month evening at Camillus Middle School that marks the beginning of our voluntary summer running schedule. Besides an easy first run, the attending runner hopefuls could expect various training information, everything from mileage targets to suggestions on running routes and requisite run garb for the hot-weather weeks ahead. Some years, overenthusiastically I loaded up the packet with extravagant explanations of training run types, 10-reasons-to-run sheets and various exhortations to log those summer miles so they would be ready come August. A few times I have prominently displayed that famous utterance from Juma Ikangaa, the 1989 NYC Marathon winner. "The will to win means nothing without the will to prepare." Other years, though, with more veteran teams, the packet was slimmer, limited to basic directives and expectations and the mileage targets assigned to different groups of runners: the returning boys and girls veterans; the new runners; the modified team members moving up to varsity. Regardless of the packet contents, I always woke to those inaugural mornings excited and optimistic.

This Packet Night, though, was thin soup. Only eleven girls showed up, none of them projected to be one of our top seven runners. As for 'fresh blood,' those neophytes who just might elevate the team's chances, only two 8th graders eligible to move up to varsity had arrived, and both had previously checked "Unsure" on the Athlete Information Sheet question about competing in the coming season.

I reminded myself that summer training is voluntary, that this was just the start and there were still school activities conflicting with my grandiose summer plans for cross-country runners. Still, there is always that early sense of 'team' based on the faces staring back. No-shows can speak as loudly of the future fate of teams as the gung-ho giddiness of attendees. A lot of average coaches who dedicate generous portions of their summer time preparing the athletes for Fall walk away from such starts with their enthusiasm dented and secretly beseeching the running gods, *just give me 5-7 dedicated core athletes and I'll figure out the rest.*

Erin had emailed earlier about her two Tuesday finals as reason for missing the evening. Terri and Sara e-mailed later with similar excuses. Pam contacted me to ask for the time of the workout, but then she never showed. Of all our potential boys front-runners for the season ahead, only Matt and Aidan occupied places on the grass. Coach and I soldiered on. I spoke briefly to the small group, then sent them on a Woods-Outer warm-up before Matt and Aidan demonstrated Rhythm Drills on the basketball court. Afterward, they walked to the outdoor amphitheater area for the evening's run.

The training trails bore evidence of our wet spring. The bottom of School Hill was a lush mushiness traced by the sunken tracks of the maintenance mowers. The heavily trafficked trail to Three Corners, a dusty, beaten highway last October was now green, rejuvenated. The Woods Loop path between the two forested sections of the course was un-mowed and overgrown. A few runners also commented on the problematic drainage at the base of the Outer Loop hill. It was saturated and sloppy and had already applied some mud stains to the legs of several runners.

The 'work' of the evening was introductory and deliberately light, two laps of the one mile Outer and Woods loops at a General Conditioning pace. I just wanted to see how they moved with that easy pace. We timed it for them, though, so they had an initial marker for how that pace felt. Knowledge of individual per mile paces also gave them the option, should they choose, to complete summer runs by time instead of distance. We then instructed to run it again, a single circuit this time, but at Steady-State pace, just so they could feel the contrast between easy and something more purposeful. One of our neophytes approached Coach G. to beg off the second effort. I came over. "What's the problem?" I asked, and the neophyte launched into a lengthy explanation of the "underwear rash" that had bothered him in a previous sports season as well. Coach G. offered an understanding nod, but I turned away to hide my smile.

His was just the start. Sally then made a strategic bathroom request, and soon after another runner copied. The others set out on their second—and final--circuit without them, and all returned except Emma. We calculated the potential places she'd gone off course, then sent Matt and Aidan, who wanted more mileage, out to search the back sections while Coach G. and I looked nearby. Walking down to Three Corners, I spied a familiar alumni face. Hunter was tallying a few miles after work and pulled up to fill me in on his current job and a recent western trip. Emma soon returned, located in the Woods Loop by Matt, where she had twisted an ankle. Coach G. directed her back to the school so she could head home to ice and elevate. We said goodbye to Hunter, gathered the runners for final drills behind the school, then called it a day. Coach and I watched them wander off into the mild spring evening and then eyed each other. Coach rolled his eyes. "It'll get better," I said, then thinking to myself, *it has too*.

July

***

After Lori decided to become a pentathlon-er during outdoor track, there was another decision she needed to make. At the end of that spring season, I had told her the same thing I discussed with so many other prospective cross-country runners. It was a well-honed speech, one I had delivered with ease to other accomplished track runners: *you have potential, but you will never know how really good you can be without the cardiovascular development of a cross-country season.* I was never sure how that invitation would be received. It had scared off a few wary souls, as though the offer was a sentence to hard labor. So, I had always added a proviso. "It's a one-year contract; try it for a season. If you don't like cross-country or you don't like what it does for your other sports seasons, then don't come back. No questions asked."

Emily, a pretty good soccer player, had listened years earlier to that same suggestion and that same offer. Then she sacrificed a season of her favorite rectangle sport, went on to cross-country and track state championships, earned state championship medals, and notched a couple of school records. She never looked back. At the end of that first school year of running, just as I had promised, I asked her one afternoon in late May if she wanted a second season of cross-country. She just smiled and nodded, as though our chat was unnecessary.

Lori, though, wasn't so easily convinced. Autumn for her meant Marching Band, a big deal in our district. Warm evenings practicing on the parking lots and playing fields surrounding the high school were her mental images of summer. Cross-Country would mean sacrificing the music she loved producing on her trumpet and the friendships forged in a tightly synchronized activity that was perfected only through long hours of daily practice. Those were powerful enticements, but now something else equally powerful was calling. So, being a product of her culture and her age, she emailed a proposal where she would not have to give up either.

It took a little time to imagine how Lori's plan for two simultaneous time-consuming activities could work. First of all, she suggested she would not be able to make our summer Team Runs because of band practices, but she promised to get in the miles. Once school started, she said, she could double up, completing our afternoon training and then filling the evening with the marching band. But, she warned, "I won't be able to participate in the Saturday Invitationals." After football games ended in late October, though, she believed she would be able to compete for a spot on the Sectional Championship team in early November. "I hope you understand how important both music and sports are to me," she closed.

Coach G. took one look at the plan and shook his head. By the end of September, he said, "She'll be overwhelmed and worn down." He also noted that all the subtractions of invested time would apparently come from cross-country. Marching band would sacrifice nothing. The next day, I emailed her.

"I applaud your willingness to take on the heavy responsibilities of trying to pursue academic excellence this coming school year while both competing in Wildcats XC and participating in Marching Band. That's the kind of determination that makes you the athlete who could take up pentathlon this spring and place 4th in the Sectional Championship. We need more athletes like you on our sports teams." Then, I listed all the reasons we could not agree to her plan.

These days, adults are advised by the so-called experts to relentlessly encourage the interests of our young adults, to help them explore, to accumulate activities and, ultimately, through such experimentation to "find themselves." We seem to have no problem with allowing them to fill their days, sunrise to sunset, with this activity and that. Some parents even take pride in how many pursuits they can cram into their child's week. These young adults are taught they should follow their instincts, their passions, that they can, most importantly, achieve anything they put their minds to. Anything is possible in America—except when it isn't. My friend and coaching colleague, Jack Reed, once remarked about the typical outcome for overscheduled students. "By committing to everything, they commit to nothing."

What the kids are less often taught is how to make hard choices, how to sacrifice one thing for another. So, I made a suggestion to Lori. "I recommend that, with help from your parents, you make a choice between Wildcats XC and Marching Band."

Days went by, and I received no reply.

***

The intent for this particular July evening Team Run on the high school track was to progress their basic foot speed with fast 200-meter intervals. First, though, came foundation-paced running to check per/mile paces. With that slower running we wanted the athletes to match their individual low-intensity paces to a perceived 'feel.' It takes practice, but such internal pace sense is important. Then, if they could only run for minutes in the mornings or evenings, they could calculate approximate distances. Only fourteen team members showed, but at least the evening's benefits would be theirs.

Matt and Erin strolled in late and nonchalantly joined the warm-up. The two had been a 'couple' since at least spring, the advantage being that if one made a Team Run, the other was almost assured to also put in an appearance. When they passed me standing near the finish line, I mentioned loudly about being on time. Both did their best pretending not to hear and melded into the circling group. And it was later, after the GC pace check and the start of the 200 meter repeats that Matt cautioned me he might not perform well this particular evening. Sometimes, runners make a habit of announcing what recent life events will likely diminish an impending practice or race effort. They hedge their bets, as though being held accountable for something they can't—or won't--achieve is the worst of fates. Matt normally set imposing standards for himself, so his proclamation caught my attention.

"Why not?"

He flashed a nervous grin. "I ran a 5k pretty hard this morning."

[216]

"You ran a hard 5k the morning of a high intensity workout? What were you thinking?"

"Well, I ran it on my treadmill at home," he said, as though that made a difference.

I just shook my head. Then he went out and proved how well you can perform summer speed-work following a morning race-paced workout.

Not very well as it turned out.

How the land....

For a long enough time, he would just bully the soil to produce. That's the way I always imagined some poor Joe and his local farmland. It was his to lose, banked heavily, the down payment on a stubborn dream. And nothing else about it, of course, would come easy—and most of it would hardly be fair. After a hundred and fifty years of cultivation, after the rolling hills and bottomlands of other parts of Camillus had offered up deposits of gypsum, plaster and clay, then grain and tobacco crops before supporting sizeable sheep herds that produced "immense quantities of wool," this poor Joe's portion of that productive swath was an irregular patchwork of shallow soils along Ike Dixon Road that served up mostly rocks. You could argue he caught the short shrift of things.

Each spring, this poor Joe's plow would have bucked against hidden boulders that he'd have to haul off to the side of the field. Then the discus would bounce over the smaller ones with a metallic whoomph as he wheeled his cantankerous Farmall back and forth in the gathering dusk. All those stones, of course, merely subtracted from the potential tonnage of the producing layer, cheating him yearly of his full crops of wheat or corn or hay. And then every spring his land was again generous to a fault with rising rocks that broke or dulled the implements he employed to wrest one more thin offering from the parsimonious soil.

Finally, he decided to cut his losses. He sold the ingrate acres to the West Genesee School district. Buildings and parking lots would soon cover some of those rocks. Others would be buried under trucked-in top-soil for playing fields. Enough land, though, would be left the way he himself had found it—belligerent, waiting to offer up annual intruders on the frost-layer express.

But that would be someone else's problem. I always imagined him standing one last time on the hill behind the eventual school and sweeping over the breath of his former tormentors with a dismissive backhand. "Fine," he'd be announcing to the fields he no longer owned, "keep your damn rocks." Then he'd smile to himself, turn, and walk away.

The runners would come later.

For years, the West Genesee cross-country harriers had been content to labor up and down the tilted fairways of the golf course bordering their high school and the nearby shopping plaza. It was a demanding 5k circuit, with hills in all the tough places and groomed scenery to match. Several

[218]

seasons after taking over the team, I even reversed the course to make it harder and added a shorter modified race line for middle school runners. Competitors would power off the fairways and finish on a playing field astride the high school to the cheers of their sparse, but loyal, fans. Once or twice, late in the season, they returned at dusk under the glare of field lights turned on for the marching band practice, rhythmic melodies rocking the runners their final tired meters.

Then, one warm spring night--not even during cross-country season--some anonymous yahoo's with cars held a party on one of the golf course greens and left it looking like four hundred moles had been invited in for a grub-eating contest. Lawyers were summoned, and the owners arrived at a brilliantly illogical conclusion—kick our cross-country teams off the property. I made the obligatory plea, asking why my runners should be punished for the transgressions of nameless others. Management, however, was not about to be persuaded by fairness or common sense. They issued their time-tested negotiations-stopper—"liability"—and we were sent packing. Could we at least occasionally run along your back fence during practices to avoid the nearby shopping mall traffic, I asked, hoping to salvage some small consolation. Nope, was the answer.

For a few spring weeks, I mentally shopped around for a place to train and compete that Fall, considering local parks or our other middle school grounds just across West Genesee Street from the high school. Nothing worked, logistically or aesthetically. Then one morning, I looked out the window of my Camillus Middle School classroom, and the light bulb finally went on. Later that day, I took a walk along the short Nature Trail through the woods behind the school. I stopped on my way back to gaze over the fallow farm fields to the west, still district property, and climbed to the top of the small hill behind our building complex. A loop cut around that field there, a trail cleared up this brushy hill here--in my mind, a course slowly began to present itself. The runners would have to be bussed over from the high school each day, but it was do-able. After mentally tracing an imaginary 5k, that night at home I sketched the first course map.

During the spring and summer months, maintenance men cut and mowed the initial rough trails I had either marked through fields or chopped out of shrub-covered hillsides. We raced that Fall on a rough but fair out-and-back course. During practices, the runners were encouraged to stop and throw off any trail rocks that had wormed their way above-ground. Mowing and foot-pounding gradually smoothed surfaces. It seemed we were home free.

Over the next four years, however, playing field constructions on the school grounds repeatedly ripped up sections of our existing competitive course. One spring, for instance, I called the then athletic director to ask why bulldozers were scrapping out our perimeter trail around the school's side lot, and he casually announced they were putting in a new soccer field. A year later, I asked the same AD why the opening loop around the school's front lawn had been buried under a leveled layer of topsoil, and he informed me they were upgrading the football field. I became adept at being ignored regarding school grounds decisions and at reconfiguring cross-country courses. Frustrated, I shelved the useless record book.

Finally, in 2006, another light bulb came on. I finagled the construction of a trail around the perimeter of our back field, a gently tilted rectangle with just a teaspoon of relief. Another competition trail section was added in 2008—the Inner Loop of that same back field—and my runners were finally liberated from everyone else's sports plans. They no longer had to run through crowds of parents watching modified soccer games or past the school's loading dock dumpster with its objective bee and wasp hazards. Except for race starts across an occasionally conscripted football practice field, the runners had this place all to themselves. Just trails and woods and seldom-used school grounds.

One summer day, I walked our newly completed Inner Loop. Coach Delsole and I had been driving over its twists and turns with our vehicles after summer team runs to help flatten the small hummocks of grass and weeds. We'd wedged out some of the bigger rocks. As I stared down the trail to where it curved into a grove of emergent birch saplings, I imagined racers that Fall angling a turn, taking aim on the woods beyond and then their long finish. Squinting into sunshine, I decided to create a new record book.

Poor Joe would have appreciated the moment.

***

Coach G. and I tallied the noticeable absences for our early-July Team Run. Some we wanted with us were on family vacations instead. That was never a problem, and we were usually notified beforehand by parents. Others, though, apparently had concocted excuses to avoid the higher velocities of our runs together. And a few, I suspect, were simply acting on the belief that you can't appreciate the hot, lazy days of summer while simultaneously training to anticipate the cool winds of Fall.

We resisted the urge to preach to the choir. They were here, after all, all eleven of them, so we sent them out on their warm-up run along the summer-etched trails, all freshly mowed. Then we met them at the soccer corner of the Outer Loop trail for final drills and instructions. The legendary distance coach, Joe Vigil, once told an audience, "You chose to be poor, average or excellent at what you do." But for many young adults, those choices are not always so distinct. Often, they themselves do not know the differences between their possible choices—or if they do, life has not yet taught them how much those differences can matter. "I wish I had…." is a reflective phrase usually reserved for a runner's later years.

After drills, though, the small crew launched into the muggy air on their first thousand-meter interval. Then, they disappeared around the far bend of Three Corners, and in the two minutes available, Coach and I mulled. We could not yet get a handle on the girls team, what they wanted, what they expected of the sport, of themselves, of each other. We wondered how many had a clear sense of purpose for the season ahead and how many were instead motivated more by obligation or some other outside influence. Vigil also wrote: "…in the end, you will train and race successfully because you want to, not because somebody else wants you to." Neither Coach nor I were inclined to push them toward self-declaration. It would have been just another source of outside influence or pressure. The 'work' of cross-country we were presenting—and their reaction to it--spoke loud enough. There are some didactic coaches who believe the opposite, and they get to work early in a season, separating, as they see it, the wheat from the chaff. *This is how we do it*, goes the edict, *this is how you must measure up.* They act as though unsure the sport itself, if faithfully pursued, will teach what needs to be taught.

Soon, down the southern side reach of our Outer Loop, where a slight dip hides the runners in their final turn, they slowly rose into view. The once bare field of years ago had grown over with emergent species that now leaned toward the taller hedge trees, creating almost a forest tunnel through which runners advanced. They crested a slight rise, silhouetted by evening light at the back end of their tunnel, then accelerated on the descent toward the finish. "Good start," I told them as they bent for a quick breath, then straightened for sips of water and to record times.

One down, four to go. Some of the newbies were already wide-eyed and questioned the number of intervals. We assured them we would monitor everyone to decide when the time had come to end. That could be five, could be four, maybe even three. We did not want to mess up their sport by making premature provisions for mediocrity.

"Alright," I instructed as they lined up for the second. "Settle into your target pace. Manageable speed is the goal and what eventually makes you racers." Heads nodded and they set off. Wendall Berry once wrote, "There is always a significant difference between knowing and believing." Some, we hoped, had begun to believe.

***

Mostly, I don't remember the things I say—or try to say—to encourage confidence or resolve in runners that lack either—or both. "Just shut up and train them," Coach Delsole once suggested we do with the chronically wary or resistant. He was right in the sense that trying to correctly gauge the inner weather of your typical young adult is, at best, a crap shoot. Mild confusion is one of the normal conditions of adolescence. So, connecting with them on the assumption of sharing understanding can be a naive undertaking. You are usually more effective managing their experiences than delivering lectures.

But there are important things to convey about the traditional truths of the sport, realities that the runners should listen to and absorb because it could save them some time and trouble. Friendly, supportive chit-chat counts for only so much. Coach D., right up to the day he'd run his last practice and moved on to other pursuits, always knew that the wisdom he'd accumulated over decades and in various coaching roles had imbued his reactions with an innate accuracy, a form of precision in sizing up athletes. He had what Daniel Kahneman called "expert intuition." He knew the difference between fluff and substance. He knew the truth about what it would take for a particular distance runner to develop and utilize his or her full potential—and who was probably game to try. Glad-handers and fakers and 70%-runners were easy for him to spot. Those were the team members who weren't really listening; they were maneuvering. Those kinds of behaviors always bothered me but Coach D. understood those gestures were not so much personal as they were simply decisions not to engage in the traditions of the sport, a circumstance where he usually considered himself mostly the messenger. He didn't waste time or lose patience with the runners who refused to listen to the messages. And that wasn't personal either, just a choice about where to put his best efforts.

My problem was that I always hoped for the breakthrough, for the transformative moment, for the light bulb to go on. Sometimes I hung in with athletes long after they'd clearly signaled they were no longer actually runners, just check marks on the attendance sheet. Coach, at least, was gracious about my eventual admissions with those failures. No I-told-you-so's. Maybe just a shrug.

"You second-guess yourself a lot," he told me once. We were ruminating after a training session, discussing a runner who did not have her heart in the game. There wasn't a cloud in the sky that particular afternoon, and the late summer temperatures were kind. Our lost runner had spent those first two weeks of start-up cross-country practices looking miserable and tortured, which she must have been. The girl was extremely talented. She had the ability to elevate the team and achieve great things, but she clearly hated nearly every minute of every practice. So we finally sat her down onet day after the work was done, and we said she should tell her parents that she had our permission to quit, that there was no sense in showing up simply to punish herself. Then, after reminding her to talk it over with the folks, we had watched her walk away. "Well, that's that," Coach had said, but I added how our permission might remove some pressure, permit a speck of insight and allow her to understand everything she was giving up. Coach nodded to show he had heard me.

We never saw her again.

***

7:04 a.m. Upper Connecticut River Valley. A few of the runners back in upstate New York were out early, pushing their morning miles in a building sweat. One problem was that they were there—and I was not. I was three hundred and twenty miles away, starring through morning haze toward New Hampshire's White Mountains and the milky bulk of Mt. Moosilauke. I was in the last days of an annual July escape with my wife to an old farmhouse outside Newbury. Coach G. had been handling the Team Runs in my absence, and, as is typical, despite the appeals of the Green Mountain State, I was itching to get home. I went back to my book and coffee, but it was already too hot to sit on the narrow, thick-planked porch facing east. I retreated inside to the cool of the kitchen with its low, big-beamed rafters.

We had it good in the valley. Back in central New York, the temperature broke 80° shortly after sunrise. By noon, the thermometer would top 90°, but with oppressive high humidity, it would feel like 105°. By 6:00 p.m.? Forget it. I had emailed the athletes the day before, alerting them if they weren't out the door for a run by 9:00 a.m., they'd lost their only chance. Our run-early-or-run-late summer mantra was reduced to a single morning option.

The meteorologists had warned us. Back in May, when everyone was complaining about the incessant rain and the chilly, cloud-ridden days, they were predicting a hot, dry summer. Well, there we were. Across the northeast, heat advisories sprouted like weeds. That hot blast, though, was forecast to last only three days before a retreat, as though the season was still practicing.

[225]

Three and a half weeks had passed. In that time, I had typed the requisite follow-up email to Lori, sending an additional note of encouragement to join, but the silence in return provided only the small consolation she apparently had at least made a decision, deciding to stick with her music commitment. Well, good for her, I thought.

One day in late July, she got in touch. "I would just like to let you know that I will be participating in the XC season this year and will sign up and start getting more training in asap. I'm not really sure what to expect from this season, since this will be my first year doing XC. However, I am excited to see what great things I can accomplish this year and to be as much of a help to our team as I can. I'm looking forward to the season!"

Rain. It rained all day. Sun afficionado's would have counted the day a loss, but coming out of a weekend mini-heat wave, rain seemed just fine. With lower temperatures and no thunderboomers stalking the area, the slow, steady precipitation was a sign the days were back to normal.

Still, suspecting that the rain would dampen more than our middle-school training trails, I was not surprised when several the runners on our annual Distance Camp roster failed to show. Not surprising, but still disappointing. Our late-July, four-evening camp served several purposes. Prospective varsity team members were encouraged to participate for an opportunity to test their training to date—a mid-summer checkup of sorts. The hope was the checkups went well and provided the group motivation to persevere. Just as important, we mimicked that feeling of the team training weeks which were finally on the horizon, not many days off. Both goals, however, were difficult to accomplish with missing faces. The camp roster, shrunken by conflicts and family vacations, included only half our prospective team members.

Our camp, though, was also open to non-team members and Modified cross-country runners. For them, the four-day agenda was an introduction to the various training types that could be useful to athletes of any sport. The associated workouts were deliberately moderate, merely samplers of the various training types. We wanted to avoid strengthening any preconceptions about running as merely torture, nor quash the dreams of any aspiring young runners with demanding hill or interval sessions. Recent running alumni usually guided the neophytes, keeping things light while entertaining them with their Wildcat anecdotes and encouragements. Coach Gangemi and I administered the harder work to our varsity runners.

The rain, however, had spoken to some of those neophytes. Of the thirteen non-team roster members, only seven huddled under our elevated walkway for introductions. And one of them announced he had to leave in forty minutes. I reminded myself that, regardless of the smaller crew, connections could be made. Some of those young faces might eventually show up on our cross-country or track rosters, remembering from our camp that they could be that eclectic personality type called a runner. That was always the hope, no matter the crowd size.

After a quick introduction with our neophyte 'campers,' I sent them out on a short GC run led by our alumni Emily and Amanda, who chatted and made introductions as they disappeared into the rainy back field. Then I walked down to Three Corners where Coach G. was staged with the varsity runners. The evening's work was an alternation run, two times the Woods/Outer loops, with the Woods Loop run at threshold pace and the Outer at GC pace. Coach Wojtaszek had shown up for his first Monday Modified Team Run, but he had no takers this rainy day and decided to tag along to watch our varsity runners go at it.

Our three top boys' runners stood around in the benign rain, joking and impatient to get started. Most of the top girls also milled about on the spongy grass. Most of them. Lori, for unknown reasons, had not signed up, even though Fall sports registrations were open on-line. She had, in fact, emailed to say she was going for an MRI the next day to rule in or rule out a stress fracture on her left leg. How, in the three weeks of recovery following outdoor track, she had managed to sustain a possible stress fracture, she did not explain. As the girls set out, I scratched my head at the prospect of losing a promising runner before she even got started. The summer weeks were creating more uncertainties than assurances.

Dale

(1962)

The slightest curl of smoke escaped from a mattress we'd propped against the wooden backstop. The discarded mattress was there to close the damage too many errant fastballs had inflicted on the aging backstop mix of rotted wood and chicken wire. Two hours into an August baseball marathon at Saunders Field, we'd been exchanging hits the whole time--and had even exchanged players. Some of them, bored waiting for grounders, scuffed the infield clean of its dry-summer weeds. The afternoon sun glared down. We sweated. By the second hour, no one had yet lofted one high enough up the left field incline to reach the old town cemetery. Legend had it, no one ever had.

"Hey!" someone yelled, noticing and pointing to the backstop. "What the?" I spotted Dale standing nearby, trying to appear innocent, glove raised to cover his smile.

By the time we rushed the backstop, tiny flames had erupted from the mattress and were threatening to jump to the dried wood. It took furious handfuls of dirt and considerable bat-beating to subdue the fire. A final gasp of smoke twisted skyward like a question mark.

"Jesus" Kenny declared nervously in the aftermath, but then most of us, Dale included, started laughing. No one, though, noticed Dale's old man already approaching from his house nearby. He lumbered toward us like a ship cutting rough water.

It was not that any earlier parental interventions could have changed anything. Dale was blessed with bravado and addicted to misdemeanor. Things happened around him by destiny. Who else, after all, could engineer the transport of old railroad ties along the trestle over the Raritan River on the opening day of fishing season—and then initiate their long and eruptive plunge into the fisherman-lined river below. We needed him to rationalize the pilfering of a church pantry cupboard for sustenance on the long walk home from a high school sports practice. *Hmmm, food for the poor*, he mumbled happily with a full mouth of canned pineapple slices. And it was Dale, after all, who convinced me to meet him on a local bridge in a sideways snowstorm one Christmas eve—just for nothing better to do.

In high school, Dale decided to become a track runner. Baseball in springtime was simply too slow. The longer distances of track, though, never intrigued him. As far as he was concerned, pacing was for patsies. The 440 yard dash, with its explosive mix of speed and power, was the only possible personality match. He'd churn down the backstretch, spikes spitting cinders, leading with the chest out and locked into that perfect one-lap symmetry of time and distance that the race embodied. Dale thoroughly enjoyed that best gift, a belief in the ultimate beauty of running fast. Fast was more than a single effort timed on a watch--or a race result. For Dale, fast was an ideal, and he continually professed and honored it in himself and others. This was also the guy who insisted he had such a firm grip on life that he would know when to let go, simply as a way to ultimately honor the gift. "The day I can't clock a fifty-three 440 anymore," he announced late one afternoon while we walked home from track practice, "is the day they should put me down like a broken horse." Dale didn't win every time he raced, but I was always envious.

We were back on the ball field and re-absorbed in the game by the time Dale's father arrived. He stomped up to the backstop, examined the charred mattress and instantly figured things out. His finger motion stopped the game abruptly, and we stood silently by as Dale slunk off the field like a pitcher who'd just been yanked in the fifth. He approached his reckoning with baseball glove flopping limply at the end of his arm. Everyone watched as Dale's old man ear-yanked him off the field and down the road toward home-jail.

"Boy!" Dale's father was yelling as he towed off his kid, "you need religion. You need religion, boy!"

August

***

August arrived, and it felt like rounding a gentle bend on our canal tow path and seeing, far away but at least in sight, a destination. The August days always gathered momentum, pulling us toward official team practices, only weeks away. Where many feel in the month's forward march a subtle and sad waning of summer, a lot of Fall sports coaches instead savor the anticipatory excitement of approaching seasons. The runners kept at their summer efforts, tallying miles and improving fitness. A positive MRI had verified Lori's mysterious stress fracture and ended her planned season. I shook my head. Another potential talent lost.

Team runs were also dwindled by final family vacations, commercial running camps and, with some, a final chance to be free of everyone else's plans. It was no matter. For the invested team members who arrived at our dog-day practices, the runs went well. Those logging their target miles continued to strengthen. They would be the ones who could absorb and benefit the most from the hard practices of late August/ September, even as we would need to modify the work of the summer drifters, those MIA's who were now fated to race their best early in the season, then trail off or stagnate because they did not have the aerobic foundation on which to build more power and speed. They were also the ones who, lacking the toughening miles of the hot months, would be prone to injuring themselves into dismay and disappointment. Still, with each team run further into August, we hoped for the return of some who had disappeared back in June. Our hopes were not rewarded. We greeted only familiar faces on Mondays and Thursdays.

One early August evening, the team run agenda was long intervals. Those showing up went hard at them, launching into the dissipating heat, pushing home and bending before taking short sips of water. Their first efforts rode on confidence, and they re-collected at our staging place with resolve. As they readied, we would sprinkle them with earned compliments: *nice finish push on that last one-- your stride looks strong--way to hang with that faster group.*

And then, with each interval, would finally come David. After a 9:37 and then a 10:34 for his thousand meters, long after all the others had pushed in, I pulled him aside. "David," I said, leaning in and intentionally filling his range of vision, "you need to run these intervals faster and without walking." David's response was to stare back blankly, so I pared the message to essential words. "Faster--and without walking."

"Faster and without walking," he repeated.

A special needs student, we were asking a lot of him. Running off others—training partners or competitors--was easier for David. His successful races proved that. But running alone in the way that required an internal sense of pace and self-awareness and self-regulatory ability—that was David's Mt. Everest. That summit would surrender slowly to his incremental efforts, after much time and effort on everyone's part. We were a couple of years into what was clearly a four-year plan.

This was, however, as good a time as any to test the powers of a great deal. "Now David," I told him, "if you run this next one faster than your first two, you will be finished. If you don't run faster, though, I will have you do one more. Do you understand?" He shook his head to indicate yes, but I wasn't so sure. "If you go faster, you will be finished," I repeated.

Coach G. sent him off again. We were watching as others churned over the final rise of our tree-hemmed leg of the Outer Loop and powered home. Suddenly, ahead of schedule, David popped into view

[233]

and pumped his way across the finish, almost four minutes faster than his second long interval. Coach and I both applauded him. "David," I said, shaking his hand, "that was much faster, and so you're finished. Tell me, how did you do it?"

David's blank stare was quickly broken by the flash of a smile, as though enjoying a good memory. "I went faster," he said, beaming.

***

Otherwise, it was a solid Team Run. August weather—those quintessential low-eighties-sunlight-poking-through-cumulus-clouds kind of days—had taken hold and would be around for almost a week. The trails were just about run-perfect, and the team members could have no gripes except perhaps about the longer grass that maintenance could not cut on their scheduled Monday because of rain. No, we were having it good. I was trying to explain the 6x800m repeats on the Inner Loop, but someone in the back of the small group had decided his lingering conversation was more important. What peeves me--and always has--is the annoyance of short attention spans. I have been around teenagers for enough years to understand they may struggle to listen. Old story. You keep the speeches short. And I have also been subjected often enough to harangues by some adults that this particular habit of youth indicates the end of civilization as we know it. That's an old story too.

There is the middle ground, and I think it is reached when I say something like, "O.K., let me have your attention please," and then wait for things to quiet down. Only sometimes it doesn't. It is that someone in the back who either decides--or has been conditioned to believe--that personal attention is a possession, not a behavior, and I'm taking away something to which he or she has a right. Those are the annoying times, good kids though they typically are. So I have to give The Speech again in a stern voice, the one about me listening to them if they are addressing me and them being expected to do the same, both of us interacting with a common courtesy that makes possible the effective transmission of information.

My speech was precisely automatic because of all the practice I get, but I was also keeping score. Tom, the new kid chatting in the back, would need to be watched. As I had told other groups and other teams at other times, unless it's a particularly egregious behavior, I seldom react to single incidents. You can't set your hair on fire over every little transgression. Patterns of behavior, however, are something else. Patterns suggest bad habits--or intent. With effort and patience, both can be changed. On rare occasions, though, with particular team members, the pattern indicates indifference. Indifference is the worst. It is the most self-defeating attitude you can encounter in athletes. Indifference is a distance that athletes open between themselves and their potential, a distance that is often impossible to close.

***

Three athletes arrived for our final summer Team Run at the canal. Three. Hell, I told Coach G.; we had cancelled other team runs with that number or less. But we decided to give these three a workout.

Justin was there, as usual. Emma arrived in her tentative manner, as usual. "Emma!" I greeted her with over-exaggeration, "How's life?" She mumbled a "Good," but I thought I detected the faintest hint of a smile, so I went on, as though addressing Coach G. "Coach, someday Emma is going to announce to me 'terrific' and then explain why." Emma had used up her smile, so she just stared.

Those two were joined by Ethan. Connie later emailed she had gone to CMS by mistake and not found us, then to the canal and somehow not found us there either. So, unofficially, the night's roster was four. Unfortunately, Connie was going on vacation the following week, our first week of team practices, so athletic policy dictated that she would be missing at least our first meet for lack of required practices. Neither she nor any others could be surprised by that since our start-up dates had been posted way back in early June.

Coach and I talked up the threshold work with the three as though addressing a full team, and then we sent them out. Only three, but each was a small show-up victory. I got to tell Ethan of his opportunity to occupy an important place on this team this fall. I made sure to compliment Justin again on the positive and productive summer he was enjoying. And I could mention to Emma about her improved arm carry as the three finished the practice with four strides. "You know," I said to Greg as they charged down toward the end of their third strider, "This season is going to be a good one for her."

With smooth, strong strides, she was making the comment look certain. Three wasn't what we wanted that evening. But three was better than two—or none. And I was in anticipatory mode. I was looking forward to standing in front of a full team on the Monday morning coming up and telling them: "Alright, here's what we've got for today."

***

The final weekend before the start of team practice, Coach and I at last knew what we would have: 16 girls, 16 boys. Any last-minute sign-ups would probably indicate indecisive team members—and potential problems. Ours would be a small but perfect balance in numbers, if not in talent or investment. Some had fallen by the wayside in the summer weeks, attending a few Team Runs, then simply not showing, their initial passions or expectations dissipating like a morning mist. Others had at first seemed 'all in' and were working hard, and then suddenly they were not, their commitments shifting. And a spectral few had attended the June pre-season meeting and were never seen or heard from again. Attrition's erasure had done its work.

Cindy was officially gone, subtracting a likely team top-5 talent. More importantly, an opportunity to introduce a young athlete to the rewarding commitment of middle-distance running was squandered—at least for the season. Gloria, that promising freshman just the year before, had never graced a Team Run all summer, and she did not sign up on-line. There would be no Jackie either, another potential top-5 team member who, after two seasons, had simply decided the rewards of cross-country insufficient to the work it demanded.

The boy's team had taken hits too. Nat had been an up-and-down runner. His ups, though, were impressive, and we hoped the sport would capture him. The parents supplied encouragement, but that wasn't enough. And one who would eventually rank high on my what-might-have been list was Gary. The year before, Gary had been

[239]

rated one of the top freshman in the section. My pitches, though, failed with Gary, who dropped any harrier ambitions to play in a fall intramural lacrosse program instead, expecting to increase his chances of winning an eventual starting position in that vaunted program. He wasn't the first--nor would he be the last—potentially superior runner to forfeit an opportunity to excel on the trails.

Others, though, were ready. Following a freshman year with too few miles of summer preparation, Aidan had languished just beyond the varsity top-7, starting strong on natural ability, then slowly sinking down the depth chart as others built speed-endurance atop superior foundations of aerobic fitness. Trying to keep up, he had pushed himself into injury and spent the second half on the sidelines, having to listen to me explain more than once exactly why he was on the sidelines. This second time around, though, he decided things would be different. His summer miles were on the chart. Justin, Mr. Dependable, had also enjoyed a strong summer. There had never been any doubt about him deliveing his best training and racing. And Matt, on a different sort of mission, had logged sixty and seventy-mile weeks as almost six hundred miles passed beneath his trainers. "I'm ready for the best season I'm ever going to have and to finish my XC Highschool career with a bang," he had emailed. The girls' front-runners had accomplished less, and I only hoped they did not then expect more. Sometimes that's the case. Everyone would begin with the miles they had banked, and both teams would arrive at Day 1 with the runners who wanted to be there. Cross-Country is a no-cut sport, but summer is its unofficial but effective try-out.

Summer had done its job.

1967

Edith was singing "Tenderly" at the clothesline while I laced up my running shoes on the back porch. "Mom, I'm going for a run," I called out, sweaty before I'd even taken a stride. It had been a summer of oven-baked New Jersey days, and we were suffering through another August scorcher. Above the pin oaks my father planted for shade ten years earlier, the afternoon sun glared down. Out front, Fairview Drive was festering with tar bubbles. Temperatures had already spiked above 90°.

My mother glanced up from her line of solar-stiffened laundry and merely smiled. She knew her approval was unnecessary. I was old enough to make my own questionable decisions.

"O.K., I'll be back," I answered her silence and took off down the gravel driveway.

My father, with a nurseryman's eye for landscapes, had constructed our oversized yellow Cape Cod house on a hill that commanded an expansive view of the surrounding Branchburg farmlands and the more distant Sourland Mountains, a gently sloping mottle of field and woods. It was a tranquil setting with only one drawback for runners. Both routes began down our hill, but both also finished up. My only choice each run was which hill to tackle on my tired return.

That afternoon I descended east, toward Neshanic Station. In those days, my somnolent hometown contained a general store, a small factory, one bar, Amerman's Lumber Yard, Orville Shurtz's arm supplies, a fire house, a store-front post office and two town bullies. For summer excitement, we'd throw stones at the passing Lehigh Valley freight trains, attempt to discover where the local girls skinny-dipped in the south branch of the Raritan River or, in my own case, schedule runs in the hottest part of the day.

At the bottom of our hill, I passed the Herforth's two collies lazing in the shade of their leaning maple tree. It was a quick push up a short rise beyond, and the road opened to a quarter mile flat bordered on the right by Stalla's farm and on the left, our good friends, the McDonald's. Heat radiated from the road, warping the outlines of mailboxes and approaching cars. Cumulus clouds drifted overhead on the slightest whiff of a breeze. I wasn't even a half mile from the house, and my feet already felt like baked dinner rolls. The Vaseline I'd slathered between my toes on some teammate's weird advice had melted away.

[241]

Sluggishly, I mounted another rise and followed Fairview Drive on its gradual descent toward the Raritan River less than a mile below. Popping tar bubbles, I passed Shurtz's farm supplies. A grizzle-faced farmer was pulling out in his battered Ford pick-up piled high with bags of fertilizer. He eyed me suspiciously, so I politely nodded and paced on, grateful for the down-sloping road. A few hundred yards further, Fairview ended abruptly at a stop sign, the farm field beyond easing down to the tree-rimmed river. I turned left, onto Pleasant Run Road, and muscled up another shallow rise where chicken hawks circled a hay field on my left. Something there had met its maker.

The road heat, meanwhile, was doing some climbing of its own, seeping up my legs, vaporizing sweat beads almost instantly. The thought did cross my mind. This would be a sensible time to turn around, jog home and enjoy a dousing with the garden hose followed by a tall glass or two of tap water. But I was a little too obstinate--and just stupid enough--so I trudged on.

That summer of '67' I was completing doubles, training early in the morning with a relaxed run, then again in the afternoon, reasoning (incorrectly) that those PM sessions during the hottest part of the day would 'toughen' me both physically and mentally. Heat, of course, is enemy #1 for the distance runner, but I lacked that information and common sense too. Common sense, though, wasn't the only thing I lacked back then. High-tech, differentiated training shoes that would nullify some of the brutalities of hot pavement were years off. And wicking was a concept for candles and room deodorizers, not shirts or shorts.

Fortunately, my lame mid-day training technique never brought me to serious grief, just some temporary misery—all of which I rationalized. With my senior cross-country season approaching, I was determined to be ready and able. When autumn returned, I wanted a key top-5 role on my squad. I wanted to impress my teammates and Coach Rogers. Mostly, I wanted, as Emerson once suggested, to be not just good, but good for something. Boiled feet and a beet-red face seemed an acceptable--maybe even a desirable-- condition in that quest.

I had nothing to lose. My first two high school years had provided conclusive proof that good wasn't going to happen for me on the football or the wrestling or the baseball teams. It took the suggestion of my sister's friend, Jack Reynolds, to break a string of sports disappointments and bring me to competitive running. I wasn't the first--and certainly not the last--athlete to fail his or her way into competitive running. It's still the irony of our sport that so many runners simply chance upon what they do best. Jack, in his relaxed northern drawl, assured me I would love running, and I had no reason not to believe him. Besides, actually being 'recruited' was a novel—and enjoyable—experience, so the spring of my sophomore year, after a winter wrestling season having my face rubbed into the mats, I traded baseball glove and cleats for running flats and joined Coach Campbell's track team.

A small percentage of the boys team members were absolute neophytes, so, by my reasoning, I had credentials. At our annual 8th grade Field Days competition in grade school, I had finished 2nd in the 'distance' event, a 600-meter run around the football field. Enough talent existed, I rationalized, for running success. Hedging their bets, my parents said nothing, which was good enough for me.

Track, however, quickly drove home the brutal truths of nature versus nurture. That first season, lacking both training and technique, I was decidedly average at best, so much so that Jack tagged me with a nickname that would stick my entire high school career. "Flash" labored through that first season sore and dismayed by the superior abilities and the cocky competitive attitudes of seasoned teammates.

I understood nothing about fast twitch/slow twitch muscle ratios and the genetic blessing of high MVO2 bestowed on the lucky few. I knew even less about properly training my energy systems. Still, if I slugged it out in the slower running groups day after day, racing the second 'JV' heats at track meets, and if I sat up front on the team bus while the veterans enjoyed their coveted places in the back, I was not discouraged. Just the opposite. Track, with its eclectic mix of body types, personalities, and motivations, was instantly attractive. And within that circus of athletes and events, the distance runners enjoyed their own special chemistry, linked by the long miles, the shared sacrifices and distinct idiosyncrasies. That sport group felt more like home than any other had, so I didn't need much convincing to sign up for Cross-Country that fall. Once there my junior year, I readily accepted a place among the other middle-distance oddballs of Somerville High School.

Up and over the rise, momentum rescued me, and I paced down toward the road's namesake, Pleasant Run Creek. For 9/10ths of the year, this benign stream meandered through farm fields and pastures toward to the Raritan River, contributing its paltry bit to a distant Atlantic Ocean. Only during spring rains did the creek ever flex its liquid muscles, and nothing but a fifty-year flood could ever liberate Pleasant Run from its constricted banks.

That wasn't happening any time soon. I plodded along the curve of the road as it mirrored the creek's gentle contours. Glancing over, summer has reduced the water course to a pathetic trickle. Gobby green algae bloomed in all the clogged backwaters, and water flies skidded across its languid, shrunken pools without the threat of bass. Roadside, in the wilting heat, I passed stubborn stalks of Queen Ann's Lace and Corn Flower poking upward, pleading a breeze. I crisscrossed the road to run in the momentary shade of large maples, hitting the halfway mark of my route, that psychological crest where turning back is no longer considered an option.

I had, in fact, limped home once from that point, stepping gingerly through hay fields on my short-cut back, a ripped heel blister sending shots of pain upward with each step. That, however, was before. One of the first things I learned from my distance brothers was that, unless you were injured or sick, finishing the run was about honoring the code. That had been made clear by my more veteran teammates. Totaling the summer miles, they'd also quickly made clear, was simply part of the job description, something you never abandoned. And if you didn't have a running partner, you ran the miles alone. Team sports have their tidy rectangles and omnipresent coaches. Runners, I learned quickly, have their unsupervised trails and roads. And runners who wanted to be good for something, my harrier teammates repeatedly confirmed with their efforts, agreed to regularly make the sacrifices--alone as often as not. They expected that. Coach Rogers expected the same. And you weren't really impressing anyone by going the extra mile. You were merely getting more of the work done.

That standard had been demonstrated the previous summer. While I trained poorly for my first cross-country season, team captains Bob Jensen and Mike Sargent had mapped out a weekly twenty-mile-long run. All summer, they and several others of the front-runners had labored through that circuit once a week. At the start of team practices in late August, they proudly beamed as they announced their efforts to Coach Rogers. Two days later he got back to them. "I drove that route the other day," Coach said. "It's only 19.7 miles."

Gruff and demanding, "Coach Robbie" commanded the Cross-Country distance runners that Campbell Platt never quite knew what to make of during spring track. Coach Platt instead handed us over to Robert Ashton, a young teacher who just happened to be a recent New Jersey AAU Cross-Country Champion. Coach Ashton could torture us with long runs into the Watchung Mountains overlooking Somerville, running backwards while commenting on our mechanics and strides. He could also pace us through 30 x 220 yards on the cinder track--just to make a point.

He accomplished it with a slightly smug smile and an easy-going, supportive nature that assumed we were tough and eager enough to absorb it all. For the most part, we were. Coach Rogers was the master of embedding expectations, and Coach Platt had eyes everywhere, spotting and supporting effort. It was Coach Ashton, however, who would guide me my senior year to the indoor track state championship mile after five weeks of home-bound mononucleosis prematurely ended my final fall cross-country season.

That, of course, would come later. At hand was the oppressive heat, more road and a hill. Always a hill. A half-mile from my point of no return, Otto Road jutted left off Pleasant Run Road, dipping down across the ever-present creek before rising into trees for a half-mile climb. Not a big deal by later standards, it was, regardless, a suck-it-up zone. I could slow on the long climb to the open fields along the crest of the hill. I knew I could even walk. Except for a passing motorist or two, no one would know. But there was, after all, the code.

Climbing the first curve away from the creek, I entered some grateful shade that came at the expense of a rising road. A short stretch of level macadam then veered left to where Otto tilted at an increasing angle. I glanced up between gulps. At the crest of the hill, not more than a quarter mile off, hot pavement would surrender to cooler dirt. Up there, I could run red-faced through a dusty runnel of poison-ivied trees and fragrant honeysuckle hedges. Up there, my pace—and my heart rate--would stabilize. Trees waiting on the downslope along the Hidden Springs settlement beyond would offer a momentary respite from the sun, and then, a mile or so still further, that last hill to my house would be, as always, the last hill. I took a deep breath, pulled the arms up and faced the hill ahead. "Just get it over," I muttered to myself.

Of course, when you're young and naive, you think you can have what you have forever. But things change. Seasons slip by. Years are added even as they are being taken away. The stride shortens, and the hills feel steeper. Sons you've yelled at and laughed with grow up and are captured by different distances. People you've loved and leaned on get old and pass away. Those honeysuckle hedges and those farm fields are eventually scraped and leveled for sidewalks and mini-mansions. The last dirt roads are paved under.

Still, echoes of everything remain--the heat, the dust under your feet, and the simple joy of covering distances. Somewhere, someone is always rising into the arc of a familiar horizon, heading home.

So you never stop searching those roads.

Fall

"*Simple does not mean easy…..*"
—Jim Brett Bartholomew,
Conscious Coaching

The ladies strolled by with their terriers. Through grateful October sunlight, their syllables fell as softly as leaves. Suddenly, a whoosh of runners thundered by on the canal tow path, and the ladies pulled themselves close, startled by the hooting high school mass of driving legs and thundering shoes. Gathering themselves, they watched the runners recede around a gradual curve while their terriers sniffed the settling dust. "Oh my," one said to the other, slowly shaking her head. "Oh my," the other one answered.

August

***

Willing to sacrifice sleep for one more late-summer evening at our Cape Vincent lake cottage, I woke 3:45 a.m., mind already running a mental movie of our first practice coming up that morning. After five minutes of opening credits, I knew that I would be lying awake for a long time that way, so I rose, pulled on shorts and sandals, said a silent goodbye to a sleeping wife, and drove slowly down the dirt driveway and into the night. Farm fields and wood lots passed dark and deep in a thick, humid air. It was too early even for the early risers, and I had only night truckers for company after I veered onto I-81 south. No distant dawn yet lightened the horizon. I passed Pulaski by 4:35 a.m. and pulled into our Syracuse house a little after five. The neighborhood was still asleep. I nodded on the couch for an hour, then rose a second time to shower and drive to Camillus Middle School.

It was a smallish group that gathered under the CMS north bridge for our 8:00 a.m. start. Chrissy wasn't there—on vacation. Erin wasn't there—still coming back from Disneyworld. Trent wasn't there—something about having to work for his dad the first week. Jessica wasn't there either—I didn't know why. Wendy wasn't there after being in the hospital with her mom until 2:00 a.m., which fortunately worked out. And Max wasn't there—no clearance on his registration. But a late sign-up—MaryAnne—showed. So did Tammi.

We had ourselves a decent weather day. I took attendance slowly so teammates could be individually recognized. Then I described

[250]

the three blocks of activity for the day. No rah-rah speech, as some might have expected. With the agenda outlined, they shuffled away on a two-trail loop warm-up before meeting at the soccer corner of our Outer Loop.

The attitude of the top girls could be summed up with a single word: wary. I was not sure why. Maybe they worried about being lectured for not coming to enough summer Team Runs or for not logging enough preparatory miles in the hot months. Maybe an isolated few wondered if I would hold a grudge against their parent's unrest and complaints of the previous Fall, unaware of my personal rule never to hold a runner responsible for their parent's behavior. The apparent reticence resisted easy explanation, so Coach G. and I put that aside and went about the business at hand.

The first business was a 3000m time trial. Some seasons, no trial is necessary. If we have the summer run logs, we know the starting points. That, however, was not this season. Questions about basic fitness were primary because too many of the weekly run totals they'd been instructed to log online were blank. So, rather than use 3-4 practices of observations to gather that information, we opted for the time trial and hard numbers.

After my final drills and instructions, Coach G. set them off. I jogged to the far corner of our Outer Loop trail where I could look down both its short hill and, over my right shoulder, the long slant of its back side. Perched there as they came around and up on the first of three loops, two things quickly became apparent. Matt was going for it, set to draw on his summer investments. He churned up the hill, chest held high, arms tucked in and elbows pumping back in sync with driving knees. He swung the corner and picked up speed down the backside, alone and driven. Mindy, too, when she came through, had no partners. She would start the season as the girls' team leader. I wasn't surprised. Whatever the drama, each summer she had been the most diligent of the girls about running preparations. Now, she had, again, already distanced herself from others who made early decisions not to match her. Pam, Tammi, and Sandy followed in their chase group.

After the rest passed through, I jogged back to the start. Coach and I watched Sara, so full of potential but so devoid of summer running, struggle by. Then Carly shuffled in after two laps. She was crying. "I can't do this," she said, sobbing, as she pulled up.

"O.K., then," I told her. "If you need to, drop out."

Dueling impulses overwhelmed her. "But I don't want to quit!" she blubbered.

"Well," I suggested, "try slowing it down, go a little further and see how you feel." With that permission, she lurched off, eventually rounding the far corner. And she did finish.

All the runners, though strung out, eventually topped the small rise of the loop's southern leg and descended to the finish. We clicked off their times. Most wore their runner's fatigue like a familiar T-shirt. They bent for breaths, then straightened to sip water and converse in low tones with each other. A few though, mimicked survival of the Bataan Death March, and I understood the trial had become more than simply a check on fitness. The check was simply to determine safe and productive starting points for training--but that implied the assumption of starting something. For a few of the runners, the trial appeared more about deciding something else. Questions now lurked behind hollow eyes and drawn faces. Dinner conversations with parents were in the offing, and one of those weighing this whole cross-country thing was likely to be our newcomer, MaryAnne. She stood off to the side, quiet with calculations of expected effort versus potential rewards already coursing through her mind.

After a short rest and an even shorter talk about the season ahead, we moved to Three Corners. The team set out on some easy general conditioning running for both recovery and more fitness building.

Matt, Aidan and Peter asked to run faster alternations instead. All three had finished the trial under control and within a half-minute of each other. They had nothing to decide except how to get better.

***

The day after our opening, MaryAnne did not return. Her legacy as a one-day team runner was confirmed by one of the girls, her decision process driven by an all too vivid memory of feelings that eventually coalesced to a single thought: *it's too hard*. But her absence had company. Tom was not there because he had to babysit his brothers and sisters. Terri was also gone because she "had to work." I merely checked them off on the attendance sheet. Their absences were familiar irritations to the expected notions of obligation, commitment and team. They were signals, however faint, to be noted for future reference. What did concern me at the moment was the absence of Tammi, even on the day that Wendy and Erin reappeared. And Jessica was MIA for a second day, so I assumed we'd lost yet another.

That afternoon the runners were to crank out some miles, though most of it would be lower intensity. Their first bout of work would be what we called segmented GC. Our Three Corners intersection of trails was a convenient staging point for those 1.5 - 2 mile intervals at general conditioning pace interspersed with quick thirty-second hits of water or simply a few deep breaths. Then Coach G. would bark out the next set of loops. Breaking it up that way offered the psychological crutch of a momentary respite in return for more mileage at better pacing. They could achieve quantity and quality in exchange for a few recovery moments that hardly affected the overall training effect. With the neophytes, it proved a good bargain, and the veterans simply ran more loops.

[254]

With a cooler morning, the shade from the bordering woods proved unnecessary, but the marshy ground that the trees sheltered were issuing an early assault of mosquitos. The runners moving in and out of the area had no real problem. It was Coach and I were forced to dig out my reserve supply of bug dope.

Before starting, we had issued a familiar and quick talk about the need to create foundational fitness and a need to sense this type of running not as tedious or boring but as a familiar movement in the bones, the instinctive motion of runners. *The easier miles*, I told them, *have to feel right, natural. When you get to that place, you have arrived as developing runners. It's that simple.* Which, of course, it isn't, as a glance at any fledging varsity or modified team will verify. But you do have to start with an ease of basic movement, whatever the pace. Everything else of the middle-distance runner's world—speed, pace changes, hill running, racing—come after, with specific modes of training. Most of the veterans possessed that ease; to others, it was foreign, at least for a while.

They racked up about forty minutes of that work, then walked their water bottles to our so-named Narnia Trail, with its short but steep hill. I pointed up. "Four hills to the top," I said. "Come down the sides and leave the middle open."

In Block Three of the morning, they were back on the flats. Another thirty minutes of lower-intensity running. The day's work ended with core drills on the school playing field. "How many miles do you think you ran today?" I asked them while they lounged before heading off home. Matt guessed about six and a half to seven. He had underestimated, but I didn't tell him by how much.

***

Tammi's father emailed me at 6:14 a.m. the morning of our third day. He wrote that Tammi had decided to quit cross-country. "She says she is going to find a job and get a car." Then he added: "It sounds to me like a teenager who is making a foolish decision, assuming that she wants to run. Last week that did appear to be her mindset."

He and I knew each other well. We had been partners several times in persuading Tammi not to abandon one season or another in the past two years, to preserve what we both believed was a positive for her. He explained she had a temporary job at the state fair, but that it did not interfere with our morning practice times. And she had not yet looked for anything more permanent during the school year. "She is supposed to see you today to explain things. She seems to be pretty determined to follow the path above. I believe she is making a mistake and will regret the decision in the future. Maybe you can get her to change her mind, but I don't think so this time." I emailed back my thanks for his notification.

There are many who will argue that it's just a sport, after all, one way among many to spend your open time. But it's more than that to the kids who want to belong to something, to actually master something, to, in fact, finally *be* something, even if for only a season or two. And that's also important to the parents who also wish something productive and positive for their son or daughter. While it's possible to argue that sport is not itself the serious business of life, what it can teach about successfully managing life *is* serious.

[256]

Coach and I watched the runners walk off from our solid and productive third day, a slow and slim parade marching toward the parking lot and rides home. Amid them, though, someone was coming the other way. Coach and I exchanged glances—and waited.

Tammi came to a stop a few feet off, squinted slightly into the sunshine but got right to the point. She said she thought it only right that she talk to us directly because—and she glanced at me—of all the days and the months and the seasons we had coached her. She said she appreciated all that time and the effort and the support. She said there had been a lot of good times, and that she loved her teammates of all those seasons. Some would remain the best friends she had. But, she explained, while the enjoyment of running remained, the desire for competitive training and racing had waned, and her team friendships had shrunk until the balance tipped. Ultimate satisfaction was lacking, and thus the primary rationale gone. All this she noted carefully, as precisely as possible.

With a thank-you, she finished as considerately as she had begun. "I appreciate you coming in, Tammi," I told her, understanding there was no longer anything to be decided. "We'll be here if anything changes. Best of luck with school." In previous seasons, even if she struggled athletically, she was still able to choose the sport for the supportive friendships it provided. But that last best reason had faded, then disappeared. Her only reason to continue would have been because others wanted her to continue, the weakest of reasons. The philosopher, James Carse, once wrote of the 'games of life' we all pursue, that "whoever *must* play *cannot play*." Tammi had come to the end of her reasons for choosing to run competitively. And she decided not to be forced to continue, to play for the desires of others.

Nodding to my offer, she turned and walked off without looking back, passing through the shadows beneath the two elevated walk bridges that linked the main school buildings, then re-emerging into the strong, late-summer light that was flooding the open parking lot beyond. There she paused and seemed to take a deep breath. Maybe she was wondering what her reasons really meant, where her decision was going to lead and if there would be regrets. Then, with a slight tilt of her shoulders, she veered and disappeared around a corner of the building.

Coach and I glanced at each other again and, for a long moment, said nothing.

Bill

I have no vivid memory of my first meeting with Bill. Soon after I started coaching varsity Cross-Country and Track, we just began to cross paths at the races and invitationals he officiated. Slim of build and distinctly bow-legged, with his starter's pistol in hand and portable microphone hung on the hip, the elderly Bill ran an efficient meet, but he also knew how and when to tweek 'the rules' in the best interests of the athletes.

And Bill never shied from a good conversation. Once, during a girls' track 3000 meter event where he was the finish line judge, we got going on the topic of runners and training during the race, so much so that when he raised his pistol to signal the gun lap, I had to quickly check my watch and discretely remind him there were still two more laps. But that was the exception, and if his attention occasionally wandered, his heart was always right there with the much younger runners he enjoyed and respected. With the progression of seasons and countless meetings, Bill's formal "afternoon coach" was eventually replaced by a cheerful "hey, Jimmy!" No one ever called me that but my mother and my wife.

Father, soldier, supportive official and athlete into his seventies. Bill tallied some personal challenges along the way, and then he made changes. That allowed him to consider those later years—the only ones left to account for—as well lived. I honestly do not know what he was thinking when, with a diagnosis of cancer, he made the decision to forego laborious medical interventions that might prolong his life. Maybe it was a simple act of faith, the way he'd learned to accept other situations—optimistically, cheerfully. Maybe, though, he was recalling his years and the rewards and the people he had enjoyed along the way—and he said to himself, 'well, that's good enough for me.' Whatever he decided, it was none of us to judge.

The autumn before he died, I bumped into Bill during a cross-country invitational he was officiating. During a break in the action, we ate a quick lunch together under bright sunshine while he brought me up to date on all his doings and winter plans. I had a team to supervise, of course. As I gobbled the last of my bagel and headed out to gather them from their cool-down run, I perfunctorily hoped he'd have a good day. Bill merely smiled, patted me on the shoulder, and said, "Jimmy, I already have."

Theirs was a slow-down strike of sorts. The runners were circling the half-mile Gilly Lake Park path on the second set of four-lap circuits: 1 lap at general conditioning pace, 1 lap at threshold, 1 lap again at general conditioning pace, then 1 lap of GC pace with 150m surge zones. The technical term for that kind of work is alternations, changing paces over a designated distance, whether short or longer. So, as Coach G. put it to pre-empt any complaints, with the sum of the jog to Gilly Lake from Camillus Middle School and then back, the maximum distance of any effort faster than 'easy' was a half mile. We sensed some weren't buying it.

They had completed the first set and then core drills during the lull. I kept them in the drills circle and built in a little more recovery with the story of one of our former runner's lead-up to Footlocker Nationals--how she'd completely changed the race strategy that had gotten her that far but would not serve her well in a national field. Front-running had been replaced with pacing in a chase pack, then using hills for moving up, with a national third place the result. The story was just a lead-in to talking about the need of each of them to discover the kind of race strategy that would work best. No one's best strategy could be everyone's best strategy—and even best strategies changed, depending. I wanted them to be thinking about that the next day in their team Time Trial. Then we had put them back on the path for set two.

Gilly Lake, once the young lifeguards have vanished back to college and visitor numbers dwindled, becomes picture perfect.

Select the right day to run the troops down there over the slight swells of Ike Dixon Road, and, while standing and watching them circle the small lake on a half-mile crushed stone path surrounded by woods and rolling fields—do that and a form of serenity settles in, as though the place has just been waiting to clear everyone for the runners. Visit on a bright and warm, early October afternoon, with drifting clouds, and you wonder why you bother training anywhere else.

"Look at that," I said to Coach G. once I noticed. Across the lake, Mindy, Erin, and Wendy were trudging along slowly, on their first GC loop of the second set. When they circled around to us, I stopped them. "Is there something wrong girls?" I asked. All three stood mute for a moment, but then Mindy spoke up. "We're tired," she said with a trace of defiance. I glanced around at the other circling runners. "Well, everyone else here is tired too. Please run the correct pace." And off they went, giving just enough extra, but no more.

Pam, Sandy and Lori, the other half of our up-front veterans, had earlier pulled ahead of the disgruntled trio and now powered along the far side of the lake. There must have been some unspoken agreement because the large group had split early into those two. What had transpired I could only guess. When Pam and her compatriots finished, we complimented them as they waited for their group-mates.

Coach G. and I talked about it after everyone had trooped back to CMS and wandered off to rides home. "Eight days," Coach G. said, referring to the early charge of Mindy that had originally impressed us. "This is the first time this season we've seen her like this." The 'this' was the resistant Mindy of last year, the wary and judgmental Mindy. I rationalized. I suggested the three of them wanted to perform well on the time trial the next day and, with institutional memory of easy pre-days, were just trying to ensure their best performances. Coach wasn't so sure. We had acknowledged to the entire team how we knew performances might be tired, but that the long-term goal of team fitness was more important than the slight weariness in a team time trial. We had three team members who apparently didn't agree.

***

The runners arrived decked out in colored T-shirts. Some wore face paint, and a few legs were decorated likewise. Several of the girls sported colored hair ribbons. As they milled, their banter was light-hearted, though a few already wore intent faces. My preparatory speech went deliberately short so they could get going on their one-hour prep before the start gun at 9:00 a.m. The sun was shining, with a comfortable temperature in the low 70's and just the occasional wisp of wind. We had a decent day for our annual Blue/Gold Race.

Each Friday before Labor Day, we would kick off the competitive season with our intramural contest on the home course. It's just a time trial, but with more hype. I would separate all the boys and girls into two teams evenly matched using previous PR's and current workout results. Everyone scored for their Blue or Gold team, so the final team points would be in the hundreds, and you could not win merely with front runners. Everyone mattered. And if we had the occasional uneven team numbers, some finish points got split. Bragging rights didn't count for much since teams change dramatically season to season, but the runners would still pack all the rivalry possible into the event. We sometimes have held a mid-summer 5k race on the course, but for the neophytes, the Blue/Gold was likely the first time they had borne down on a 5k with something important at stake--the winning team lined up first for food at the school cafeteria Team Brunch line after the race. No one, though, has ever shown up with a "Will race for Food" T-shirt.

While the runners completed warm-ups, Coach G. and I checked logistics. We had conscripted our injured runners to hand out finish cards and then tally the all-important final team scores. Coach G. would click off finish times while I moved around the back fields with a walkie-talkie to monitor runner safety and cheer on the troops. Aside from the large orange cones that delineated our school grounds loop turns, nothing else on the course was marked like a regular league meet. The team members were expected to know it by heart. The runner's competition maxim--*know thy course*—had been discussed more than once.

By the time the teams assembled in front of the start line for their pre-race squad cheers, a small crowd of faithful parents and family members had gathered along the narrow macadam drive behind the school. Coach G. brought the runners to the line as I climbed the hill behind the school. I wanted to photograph the start before disappearing into the back trails. The horn sounded and they shot off. From up high, they looked like charging figurines in that old electric football game from the late fifties. They veered around the first cone and pumped up the rise along Ike Dixon Road, the starting clump of runners stretching out like pulled toffee. *We're into it now*, I thought.

With a last glance over my shoulder at the leaders powering along an elevated shelf of grass above a baseball field, I descended a trail to the Outer Loop and took station at Three Corners. It wasn't long before the leaders came charging down the Connector Trail from the school grounds and powered toward me. No surprises. Matt was going for it again and had already opened a sizeable gap on the others. The year before, he had done the same, finishing over two minutes ahead of that promising freshman who had deserted us for lacrosse's 'Fall Ball.'

Another freshman, though, had taken his place. Peter was leading the small band of pursuers who soon streamed past me, dipping down beneath the canopy of trees that separated Three Corners from the Ike Dixon field and the Woods Loop. The others churned through. Not surprisingly, Mindy zoomed by, ahead of the other girls, powered by the strength of her summer miles. She would finish a full minute ahead of Pam and eighth overall in the race. I cheered them on, jogged several hundred meters to catch glimpses of some exiting the Woods Loop and then, after that, retraced my steps to where they entered our difficult, last-added trail, the half mile Inner Loop.

Years before, when Coach Delsole and I had marked out the last needed addition for our secluded 5k, the field had been nothing more than grass with the occasional emergent seedlings or shrubs. Decades later, the runners you could once visually follow around it from a viewpoint on the school hill were now concealed by groves of birches and other succession species vying to reclaim the field. Only our mowed trails staunched their total advance, creating in spots, a shaded trail.

The Inner Loop usually proved the crux of the course for runners. Its difficult and sinuous route contrasts with the rectangular dimensions of the sister Outer Loop. Runners reach the two mile mark near the end of the loop, where it climbs a spine of open ground in the field. At that point, the runners can see the Woods Loop they must repeat clockwise and, across the overgrown field, the steep Amphitheater Hill climb that waits and will still leave them with a half mile to the finish. Our Inner Loop usually separates the runners willing to push on at that point of accumulating fatigue from the others whose inner voice counsels them to slow and reserve energy. Go or slow--races between battling competitors are often won on that mid-race section. Push the Inner Loop is a mantra for our runners.

Matt ran the loop strong, as did the chase pack following him and most of the girls' veterans. Some of the neophytes who lacked summer fitness and race experience, however, came down the Inner Loop's exit hill looking wide-eyed and exhausted. They were still a long way from the finish, and they knew it.

Ten minutes after Matt crossed the finish, the teams milled around the chute area and recovered as the last runners trudged home

[265]

to claps and cheers. Matt had come through with one of the all-time top-10 Blue/Gold efforts, and Peter cruised in second. His older brother was further off in fourth, but with a promising start. In the middle school cafeteria after team cool-downs, they congregated at tables, gabbing it up and starring at the sumptuous brunch set out by our parents group. Coach and I re-checked the final tally and, after a few comments on good efforts, announced the 171-180 score. Cheers erupted on the gold squad as they lined up for first dibs on the feast. Our season was officially underway.

September

***

Early in the morning, from the open tailgate of my Forrester parked out on the basketball court, I watched as they wandered in and congregated beneath the walkway-bridge. And then, as though enveloped in a glass bubble, they milled around there blissfully, despite my calls for them to come over. These were adolescents well practiced in ignoring adult decibel levels. Finally, I got David's attention. He meandered over, and I sent him back to get the others. I watched him stop halfway and bellow with unaccustomed authority, "Girls! Come over!" The girls roused themselves from their conversations, picked up bags and trudged toward me. The boys finally took the visual cue and followed. Practice began under bright sunshine.

It was their last day of freedom, so I had some empathy. Tomorrow they'd all plunge into the hectic, heady atmosphere of the modern American high school, this one replete with anticipatory teachers, some more versed in high school opening days than others. At that moment, in fact, the teachers were assembled in the high school auditorium listening to renditions by the school chorale, of which Erin was a member and thus absent. A few sicknesses, a few injured runners and one other conflict had shrunk our group, but not by much.

This day would be easy, the first practice we'd taken the foot off the accelerator. Coach G. was away at his school workshop day, listening to Erin. Thanks to retirement, I decided to stick with a morning practice. Their rush back into the school world the next day would include our first league meet. So, on the pre-race short agenda was a general conditioning run, a small amount of threshold pacing, uniform handouts and finally some strides and sprints on the school fields for a touch of speedwork and 'start practice.'

Everything went well until the strides at the end. Despite my warnings, athletes jumped the command and had to drop for the mandatory push-ups while the others chuckled and joked. It was all in good fun but with a point: pay attention. "It would be truly embarrassing," I reminded them, "to false start in a 5k cross-country race." Aidan had been the one to false-start with two others, and they all cranked out their push-ups. Then, Aidan false-started again, coming up with a sheepish grin after dropping for another set of ten. And then, almost as though he had simply lost all short-term memory, he jumped the command a third time. The others simply hooted, and Aidan went into that mental record book of curious and arcane Wildcat XC firsts.

***

The athletes whizzed through a full schedule of shortened first-day classes, completing an entire school day in half the time. Then they returned at 3:00 p.m. to board our Team Bus. Nothing, though, about our afternoon would be compressed. We were going to start the school year off with a league meet against the #1 state-ranked Fayetteville-Manlius boys and girls teams.

When we arrived at their hilltop high school, a place perfectly situated to catch just about every wind gust visiting the area, there were no home athletes and no finish chute where it had always been. The athletes dropped their backpacks against a side of the building near the tennis courts, and I went looking. Reaching the lip of the short but steep terrace hill that once served as the finish to their course, I peered down. There, nested beside the boundary trees below, was the chute. Nearby, two large cones marked the start. Our boys had already headed out on their warm-up, but I walked back, gathered the girls, and we trudged down the hill to find a new team spot on the grass off the side of the start-line. One of top F-M girls came walking by and stopped. Phoebe, who recognized me, said, "The course has been totally changed." I smiled. "Yes, I guess so. No more finish hill." She described to our girls the general shape of the new course. We thanked her, and she took off with several teammates to complete their 'warm-up,' which was really a full-blown workout. The race against us would be their day's 'finisher.' Neither I nor the runners took that as an insult, simply an indicator of the quality of their program. I had already told our runners to not only race hard that day but to observe. "Watch what they do both before and after the race," I had instructed both teams, needing to say no more. Great teams are neither mysteries nor mythologies. They are typically a mixture of very athletic individuals and the ways in which they agree to arrange their lives in order to maximize their talents and skills.

An hour and a half later, both our teams had taken their beatings. Matt and Peter placed 2nd and 5th against their pre-fatigued competitors to create a respectable 21-40 loss. Our girls, without the benefit of a team front-runner, were swept 15-50, but Mindy had cracked the top-10 with the third fastest per mile average of her career. Pam, with the eleventh spot had accomplished the same. They were not alone. Most of the runners on both our teams produced dramatic improvements in their time-trial mile averages. Our emphasis on building foundational fitness seemed to be working. Coach G. and I were satisfied with the efforts and, by the conversations with athletes as they snacked on apre-race snacks, most of them shared that conclusion. Everyone boarded the team bus for home thinking it was a decent enough start. Not great, but good enough.

With Coach G. away three days at a good friend's wedding, I gave the troops their marching orders for our Friday pre-race day: six loops of general conditioning running, with each loop containing 30-45 seconds of 'up,' a variant fartlek run of sorts. Then they would complete eight minutes of threshold around the playing fields before two strides and two sprints. Just enough and not too much. Their opening big meet of the season, the VVS Invitational, was the following day. The weather, of late summer vintage, felt intoxicating, with low 70's and columns of cumulus marching through on slight winds, rhythmically interrupting the gentle sunlight.

Once my runners left for their loops, I watched the modified coaches working their runners—my first chance of the season to check on them. Coach Wojtaszek was leading them through drills, and I liked what I saw. Most noticeable was their numbers, probably fifty boys and girls runners total. Less evident, but no less exciting was spotting signs of athleticism in the young runners, spying who displayed a rapid turn-over in his or her stride, who displayed that bounce, that "bong" in the drills that gave evidence of fast-twitch muscles and efficient energy storage in the legs. I scanned for those who simply looked the part of middle-distance runners. There were more than a few, and Coach O'Keefe, standing with me, pointed out several team members she thought had great potential. The group was the visual payoff of our planning at the end of last year's disappointing seasons. The goals had been set and the strategies followed to re-shape and re-invigorate the modified program, a program that, through

[272]

several years of revolving or ineffectual coaching, had withered and weakened. With Coach W. and Coach O. back, a sense of order and continuity had been restored. There was, of course, no shortage of what you'd expect on a modified team, the goofy and the gawky but enthusiastic middle-schoolers still learning how to listen. But the hidden gems were motoring amongst them, and I thought to myself, *this is what I've wanted to see.*

***

Coach P. volunteered to help out, and climbed about the team bus to our Vernon-Verona-Sherrill Invitational. Along the Thruway, central New York passed by under a sky locked down with clouds, some of them threatening, though the windows never streaked with rain. A few of the runners chatted quietly. Others stared silently at the passing scenery. Of them all, only Sarah would be unable to compete due to injury. The teams seemed confident as we circled into the school's side entrance, unloaded and trudged to the team tent area to set up. It would be a short day, with both varsity and JV runners competing in combined races— and with the girls and boys race starts separated by less than an hour and a half. The meet director had placed us in the third of four sections of races, and the meet lottery had awarded us start box #1, a straight shot to the first turn of the course. After the team tent went up, some runners hustled off, hunting their first prize of the day, meet T-shirts at the concession stand. A few parents arrived and mingled—but they would keep discrete distances once the teams began their focused one-hour countdowns, what we called 'getting in the bubble.' The parents knew the expectation and all the reasons.

In the years when VVS also hosts the November sectional championship, their early season invitational provides a form of runners' symmetry, big-meet bookends to the team season where an optimistic start in early September later reaches a November closure that is either satisfying or disappointing or, more commonly, some mixture of both. The runners, though, were not considering seasonal symmetry, just the immediate task ahead.

Shortly before their race, as the girls changed to spikes, I saw Emma struggling with hers. She was trying to untie a massive knot that had dried tight as wood. So I stepped over. Understanding, she wordlessly handed over the mess. The others were busy pinning bibs and hip numbers as I unraveled the knot and handed back the shoe. Then I circulated through the tent, reminding the girls to leave time for final threshold running before reporting to the line. I noticed Emma again. Now she was struggling to attach her bib number, so I whispered to Erin, who sidled over and quietly offered help. The girls finished their preparations, gathered, and jogged together to their box on the start line, joining a busy throng of warming runners, coaches and spectators. Ten minutes later, after strides, sprints, a team cheer and the start gun, the Wildcats were disappearing into the back woods amid a small legion of charging competitors and cheering spectators.

From a familiar spot near the back field of the course, I watched them pass three times. When they first emerged from the woods and flew by near the mile mark, Mindy, as expected, came through our lead runner. Pam, though, paced not far off. Both bore intently on, turning back into the woods, and were followed seconds later by Wendy, Sandy and Lori, all tucked into clumps of competitors. I jogged to a new position, catching them again as they quickly circled back out of the wood and around the looming water tower, dropping down into the back field loop. My shouts mixed with mental calculations. A quick glance indicated they were in trouble against the Central Square team, who matched up ahead of each of our top five runners. I shouted at all of them to move up, to push harder, then I did another quick count as they exited the short field loop and headed a last time into the woods. Tammi and Pam were moving strongly, but Wendy, her turnover slowed and laborious, was paying for a first half raced too fast. Lori, lacking race experience, had grown tentative in the

[275]

middle mile and fallen back. Erin simply seemed to be struggling, having one of those 'bad days.' My jog up to the final rise overlooking the stadium and the closing loop was short, and fans and coaches had already lined both sides of the course. Cheers erupted as the lead runners swung into sight and labored up the rise. Cameras and cell phones busily preserved the accumulated fatigue in the runners. The crowd cheered on all of them. I scanned the field, and after our lead runners had passed, I projected second place for the girls. Time had run out for individual moves that could make a difference. I jogged toward the finish paddock to greet our weary crew.

It was only later, when our team was announced as the winners of our third race, that I heard six of the lead runners had somehow gone off course in the final meters of the finish loop and been disqualified. Just far enough back, and disciplined enough not to follow, none of our leaders suffered that fate and were moved up in the finish order. Tammi and Pam earned top-5 finishes. Our critical scoring fifth runner crossed in sixteenth for the team win. The girls celebrated. Many factors converge to create competent races, but the runner's maxim, know thy course, is always on top of the list.

The boys race came up quickly, and they gathered at their start line position, exchanging remarks and fist-bumps. They had completed their sequence of stride and sprint-outs and were already steeled to the presence of a formidable McQuaid team ranked thirteenth in the state. But after a quick chat with the McQuaid coach, I had some news for them. "Guys, I just want you to know that McQuaid is running its JV team today here. Their varsity squad is at a meet in Ohio. Go out and win this." Which is what they did. With Matt and Peter finishing 1-2—and four of our runners placing in the top-20—they beat their closest competitor by 64 points.

Both teams later collected their team first place trophies. Parents hugged their runners and offered me congratulations. I smiled my thanks but knew the most important results would come later, after Race #4, when the total meet merge would be calculated by Leonetiming. With those later results, the girls would rank ninth in their forty-four team field and the boys the same of fifty-nine teams entered. I wanted better. But at the moment, they took turns holding their trophies and posing for photographs. Coach P. and I were discussing the work ahead when the boys JV results, also calculated from the total field by Leonetiming, were announced. Justin heard himself declared the individual winner of that race within a race. For two seasons, he had labored for what he really wanted, a team top-7 varsity spot. But he wasn't about to waste a perfectly good moment. He shot up from his sitting spot in the team tent, arms poked upright as though signaling touchdown. "Number one!" he shouted to the wild applause of teammates, "Yes!"

***

Soft sun and mild temperatures celebrated our first home league meet. Summer was surrendering graciously--and on time. The contest had drawn probably the largest group of spectators in the past eight years. They milled about—mothers, fathers, grandmothers, a person with a dog sporting a "West Genesee" kerchief around its neck, little brothers and sisters that raced through the crowd, people seated comfortably in their portable lawn chairs on the macadam drive astride the middle school—all enjoying the meteorological parting gift. Some estimated the crowd at three to four hundred. Liverpool and their faithful followers had certainly swelled the numbers.

I stood near the finish with several of our girls' top runners. They had just turned in their place cards and were sipping water after a draining race, one contested in the early going but finally dominated by Liverpool's #5 state-ranked team. Mindy had pushed hard with the Liverpool front pack and been in third place coming over Amphitheater Hill and into the final eight hundred meters. But she was caught along The Terrace by one of her competitors and then, as they curved down across the school field for the final sprint finish, by two more. It was a too-familiar sight, her difficulty at summoning fast-twitch muscles for a strong finish. Watching, I simply sighed. Mindy certainly wanted to be faster at those moments, but she had also resisted all my past suggestions to run the track seasons that might not make her a sprint demon but would at least improve her basic foot speed. Other sports or other activities had been more important. Finishing close behind Mindy was Pam. She had raced thirty to forty meters off the lead pack—a distance conceded early in the race—then slowly closed in the final half mile. She pushed the pace late, with the finish in sight, when she felt safer to take the chance. But she was too far back, so hers was another missed opportunity.

Most people want to believe coaching is just a matter of taking the time and finding the right method to "reach" an athlete, especially young athletes. Create the incentives, they say, that match the aspirations. Be patient and persevere with the positive. By those beliefs, coaches who can't channel the desire or find a way to inspire an athlete are said to have failed, not the athlete. But sometimes that is a simplification, the dismissal of an athlete's responsibility to acquire that most difficult of human attributes—the ability to be accountable. Coach Jensen once told the story of a track and field team member, a talented kid, who had trouble making practices. He would come a few days, then miss a day with some lame excuse or no excuse at all. Coach J. tried everything he knew to rouse some sense of investment, some commitment, in the athlete. He checked to make sure there was nothing outside of sports and school causing the problem. There wasn't, and nothing was working. Weekly, the athlete was making a charade of what it meant to be a contributing team member--and he was affecting the efforts of his teammates. So, one day after missing yet another practice, the athlete showed up and Coach pulled him aside. "Here's what we're going to do," Coach told him. "I want you to take two weeks off—then quit." There are, after all, limits.

With making practices, Pam was as dependable as they come, but she made other decisions. One of those was about how many risks she was willing to take in practices and races, which is another way of saying how much fatigue she was willing to endure. Whenever runners launch into that unknown, an athletic venture beyond their natural homeostatic preservation of self, it takes both faith and desire. Somewhere, somehow, they have mustered the resolve to discover what's over the horizon of their more familiar efforts. It's the moment when the regulatory voices reminding them of *what I like or what I choose to manage are*—for at least a short time— ignored. They take the risk and plunge ahead. When we talked about it, I usually reminded Pam of the races when she had thrown caution to the wind, those inspiring efforts when she had wanted a race badly enough to push earlier, to take risks. Personal records and important qualifications had always been the result, but they never convinced her to regularly tap her full potential. She remained a cautious racer, starting conservatively, holding back in the middle of competitions, then coming stronger at the end with distances to competitors impossible to close.

"You know," I said to her privately after the race, away from the others, "if you'd gone out just a little faster the first mile, if you had kept that gap smaller, you would have passed that entire group coming in. You're that strong." Pam, as always, listened politely, but she didn't seem to be seriously considering the possibility. She had, after all, just raced her all-time PR on the home course and finished seventh in a race against a top state team. That, she might have argued, was effort enough. "I guess you are hard-headed that way," I said, but with a smile. Ours by then was a tacit understanding. Pam was going to stay cautious, but she also knew I would keep trying. So she simply smiled back.

***

Two thirds of the way through our long-interval workout around the indoor CMS hallway oval, as the athletes bent over for a breath on the windowed bridge that connects the main building with the gym and cafeteria areas, the heavens outside opened and delivered a lashing rain. Earlier in the afternoon, after checking the ominous weather radar, I had suspected trouble and moved the workout inside. The runners had silently appreciated that decision. Following a hard opening mile in the snug hallways, they logged three 4-lapper 1000m repeats while heavy rains moved in and lashed our glass-paneled bridge. As their chests heaved before the final mile effort, thunder rumbled, which meant lightning somewhere. Soon, all the other outdoor teams—soccer, football, modified cross-country—began straggling into the building, athletes hunched like soaked rats off a sunken ship.

The biggest problem for our runners then became not the grueling mile interval left, but water tracked in by other sports refugees. Slipping on a corner wet spot could be disastrous, so we shouted the soggy players off to the safe side of the hall, actually forming a human guardrail with myself and some of our injured athletes sitting out the practice. I grabbed a mop from the janitor's closet and quickly dried one or two wet spots. Then I positioned myself by the entrance corner of our oval to play cop with modified athletes now waiting for rides home, their practices abruptly cancelled. Coach G. set our runners off on their final mile. It was a straightforward question we had posed to them beforehand: could they suck it up and hold their first mile pace in their second bookend one? Did they have that left in them?

They circled while I shouted some bewildered bystanders away from the hall corners. The music director, holding practice in the cafeteria, came out to complain about the noise. I had runner safety on my mind, so I ignored him. Matt bore through and crossed the finish cone first, wobbling listlessly off to the safe side of the hall. The rest streamed in, at least half of them having beaten their opening mile time. Sandy and Lori went down on all fours, heaving for air. Clustered near the front door, a small group of middle school athletes stared wide-eyed at the two of them, as though they'd just seen a ghost.

***

Rumpled, dirty-gray clouds like old sheets shrouded our discrete, last-day escape of September. Erratic spatters of rain, simply because of safety issues, had nixed my idea of a long run along the country roads and farm fields northwest of the school. Another time for that, I thought, maybe some Indian Summer afternoon in early October when sunshine paints the fall foliage and livens the blanched cornfields waiting harvest.

The teams gathered under the school bridge in the annoying drizzle. Our Monday practice marked more than the end of a month. We had concluded the August and September weeks that I explained at the beginning of team practices, the unwelcome ones dedicated to developing the basic aerobic fitness too many had neglected in June and July. Time was running out for some, but those team members who would qualify to move on to the Sectional Championship in November still had a month and a half to their season. Maybe time enough.

On the drive to practice, with a mood matched to meteorology, I had thought about what was already lost to this season. For too many, that had been the absence of maximal summer preparation. But there were bigger issues. Three of our expected top-7 girls' runners, for their own reasons, had decided cross-country was no longer worth their efforts and left the team. Cindy, another potential top performer, was lost to her non-sport summer injury. For the girls team, the season had been one with too many subtractions. The same, though, was true on the boys' side. Several with talent had simply declared *no mas* even before the summer training. Coaches always begin a season with two questions that must be answered. The first comes as naturally as breathing: *What have we got?* The answer to that must be objectively honest, and it must address not only the presence of realized and potential talents, but the attitudes and demeanors and desires of the runners who do, in fact, show up. The second question requires some forward thinking, as well as a sense of adventure: *What can we do with what we have?* The question sits in front of you every afternoon, waiting to be answered.

The McQuaid Invitational, the midpoint in our uncertain season, was two days behind us. Both teams had been slotted into the large schools seeded races that were ladened with exceptional schools. Both our teams had given it their best shot, not placing as high as I'd hoped, but not finishing last either. The boys, young and evolving, with two freshman and a sophomore in their top-5, had not even raced a top-10 West Genesee team time on the McQuaid three-mile course. It was easy, though, to speculate success in their future. The girls' team time, however, was the slowest ever. Though I never brought up the fact, I felt bad about that simply because they deserved better. Since stepping out of an unaccomplished summer, most of the girls had, in fact, worked hard and more effectively. Like the boys, they could envision stronger future teams if they wanted to look ahead. Their girls modified counterparts had captured second place with a 7th grader racing to 2nd individually and with eight girls in the top-50 of their large 240 runner field, more than any of the competitors. A front-runner plus strength in numbers spelled good things for the future of our girls' varsity team. If all those young runners brought their talents up to the varsity ranks, good things were going to happen. But that was the future I had the luxury to contemplate. My team members were living in the present.

So, the varsity members huddled under the bridge as rain continued to fall and waited for the inevitable speech they expected--judgment on their Saturday results. "I was going to talk a little about your effort levels at McQuaid," I said to them, noting downturned eyes, "but I really have nothing to say. You're fine. Your level of effort right now is fine. You're giving it all you have. Just keep doing that." Then, spying several relieved faces, I sent them out on the warmup.

Pat

More often than not, whenever I held an impromptu meeting with my runners during cross-country practice, it wouldn't be long before I wasn't the only one talking. Another voice would invariably bubble up in the back of the assembled squad, and it was always the same voice. So I would simply surrender the airwaves, and soon, noticing the conspiracy of silence and turned heads, the offender would quiet himself while swallowed chuckles rippled through the group. They knew what was coming next. I'd drop a deep breath and shake my head. "Pat, come stand by me." Dutifully, but always smirking, Pat would mosey up and plant himself by my left shoulder, where he'd remain perched, quiet and compliant as clay, while I finished whatever I needed to say to the others.

Pat and I discussed this breach of courtesy, but it never changed. It became, in fact, a routine as predictable and reassuring as drills and daily attendance. We'd be assembled aside a farm field or grouped on a trail rimmed by September golden-rod or tucked into the far-flung corner of some frosted school grounds. The crisp, evanescent autumn season would be streaming by us, days twisting off the calendar like sad leaves. I would be talking about this or that thing concerning their running lives. And Pat would always wind up there beside me, smiling, without an apparent care in the world.

October

***

The first day of October was a hot one—and not even by relative standards. It was hot, 86° with a 'feels like' of 92°. I had to pull out the Heat Index guidelines to review our procedures and then reassure the athletes, assembled in the shade under the crossing bridge, of the precautions we would follow. The year before, I had been criticized by some over-protective parents for pushing their kids "too hard" in hot weather--even though we had followed those same guidelines. I didn't need that conversation again. This Monday afternoon would be the last grand gesture of a calendar-gone summer, so we bowed to its admirable effort by modifying the length of the workout and increasing recovery stops.

They headed out to our staging area in shorts and T-shirts. Jeremy lugged that ridiculously huge jug of his which held enough water to put out a small brush fire. Once they returned from a shortened warm-up run, what I noticed immediately was that freshman Mike was decked out in thick dark sweatpants, unlike all the others relaxed in their summer garb. He caught my cross-eyed stare.

"I didn't pack my shorts," he explained meekly, probably having gone all-in on my previous warnings about the cooler temperatures in the weeks ahead.

"Didn't you check the weather report for today?" was the obvious question.

Sweaty Mike replied with a quiet no, then tilted his head to one side. "Rookie mistake, coach," he said with a disarming dose of chagrin.

[288]

I laughed. Mike wasn't offended because he knew he was off the hook. I was still laughing when Coach G. meandered over to see what the joke was all about.

***

The preternatural heat of early week slipped off as quickly and quietly as it had arrived, like a thief. A more realistic wet and miserable rain settled in the day after Mike's clothing faux pax. By the time I drove through the Sims Store lot at Erie Canal Park to the covered pavilion, the rainfall had slacked. Every slight wind gust, though, shook heavy raindrops from the trees that kerplunked loudly against the shelter's aluminum roof. For all the gloom, this was the place of choice for our practice. Better they pace the absorbent tow path with its available pavilion shelter than slip and slide around the CMS rain-soaked trails, accomplishing little and smearing the paths down in the process. I pulled on rain pants and an extra layer. When the shuttle bus pulled in and disgorged the team, the rain had subsided, leaving a cool, wet and deserted canal. No dog walkers or bikers in sight.

The runners dropped their dual, counterbalanced bags--school and running--on the picnic tables and continued their conversations. I took a mental headcount. Mindy and Wendy were missing. I assumed Mindy had waited to drive Wendy over after her arrival from a technical school she attended in the afternoons. But even after the team returned from their mile 'Shack-n-back' warm-up, the two had not arrived. So, I wondered.

Since late September, Coach G. had noticed it first. He had a good eye; he caught many of the inconspicuous and transitory behaviors of our runners at their sport, moments easily overlooked but that were signals. He described some moments when a gregarious group of

[290]

girls chit-chatted before a practice, and Mindy would be standing off to one side, uninvolved. There were also the moments when she left practices by herself while others stood around to gab or walk off together. Coach noticed her sitting alone on the team bus rides to meets. Mindy had never been considered outgoing, but it was still his impression, Coach said, that she seemed more withdrawn from others than before. Something was going on.

What we did know was that over those past weeks, she had missed at least a practice a week, sometimes two. Her mother had sent typically terse, one-sentence e-mails to inform me of her absence due to "an appointment." No other information, as though we had no need to know. The appointments, however, were adding up and her attendance average was dropping. She was missing required practices and important training just at the time we moved toward final invitationals and the championship races.

Her teammates, of course, knew why, and one told me that Mindy was receiving tutoring. That simply struck me as odd. Normally, we bend or waive team rules to accommodate any significant academic needs. But that clearly wasn't the case. Mindy was one of the brightest students in her grade. Tutoring had obviously been arranged for some other purpose, one the parents never bothered to communicate to us--and the choice of conflicting times seemed deliberate. It was not the first time she had gone MIA from important practices. The year before, she had missed several team days for a school function. When I confronted her about that, she claimed the Homecoming Committee was just as important as our team training. Questioning her daughter's decision earned me the ire of her mother and might have precipitated that mom's campaign to have me fired. This latest string of absences seemed more of the same.

That morning of our canal practice, after our voluntary A.M. lifting session attended by a small core of runners, I had told Pam and Sandy what Coach G. had noted recently and straightforwardly asked them if there was any issue involving Mindy. They shook their heads no and headed off to prepare for school. That was still on my mind as I sent the runners out on their down and back four-mile GC run. Minutes after they left, Mindy and Wendy arrived. "We were waiting to see the trainer. It was crowded," they explained. I told them to head out and group up with the others when they met them coming back. They disappeared around a bend in the tow path.

***

By Friday, the day after our canal run, only winter had failed to make a visit. Heat, cold rain, sun, wind--we had seen everything else. The day's drab clouds had at last been squeezed almost dry. Intermittent drizzles were their final offerings as the troops assembled near the Woods side of the Inner Loop. With no Saturday invitational this week, I told them, "Time to hammer." The work was six times 800 meters running counterclockwise on that sinuous loop, which meant starting up its short hill and into the lowering sun. A one-to-one recovery was assigned each effort. Instinctively, the runners began to group. "When it gets hard…," I announced loudly. "Push harder," one of the guys answered, finishing my sentence. Some of them were twitchy, ready to go at it. Some were not. Unfortunately, some who might have shined that afternoon were simply not there. One by one, Coach G. set off the groups.

It is true—at least to me--that if you know your runners well, their likes and dislikes, their moods and their habits and, most importantly, their competitiveness—if you know those attributes, then you can probably imagine watching a workout like this even if you never attend. The interval watch times speak their personalities and their inclinations toward effort, aspects of individuals you have watched countless times. The slow, cautious starts, the slower times in the middle intervals, the fast finishes when there's nothing more to chance or the drop-off times of the less fit. Those number scenarios recorded on paper all have faces attached to them, though it's never our job to simply look at times, and the times are never the full story.

When they launched out on the first interval, the temperature hovered around fifty and the winds slanted west-northwest at ten miles per hour. The trail surface was firm because it sheds water better than our other trails. And that drizzle, when it occurred, was not really a problem.

Peter made the obligatory stab at holding with Matt, but his gambit only worked for one interval. What really caught my eye was watching Aidan and Andy punch in times faster than the front two. And they did it again on their second loop. But they had pushed to their maximum and settled into a groove for the third and fourth while Peter and Matt pushed the pedal down ever so slightly, expertly attuned to their internal signals that told them they were good to go. Eight seconds faster on the second than the first for Matt, then fourteen seconds faster, then ten. For a well-trained and mentally disciplined distance runner, he was living the dream. Under control and going negative.

Then it got harder, that moment with this type of work when feeling fails as an accurate estimator of pace. The further in, the harder you work for fewer seconds won. And sometimes you don't win seconds; you just hold on to what you have. In this type of practice, it was that moment—the interval *before* the last one—when workouts for the inexperienced or the unfit can falter or even blow up. "Push this interval," we reminded them again. "You know you will push the last one." Peter dug in, though his time increased slightly on the fifth. Matt, though, dropped still another second. The question then became the same for everyone else as they queued for their last circuits. How well would they close? Had the proper work trained some of those fast-twitch muscles to be recruitable for the last effort? Had the willpower been inculcated that could force the matter? Every one of the top-10 boys dropped their times. Nine ran their fastest interval of the afternoon. All of them bent over, gasping oxygen and starring at the ground between their feet.

Not to miss out on the fun, Pam, Mindy, and Erin formed a trio of precise practitioners of the negative. They did the boys one better. They were three seconds faster on the second interval. Then minus four seconds on the third, then minus three, then minus five and, finally, minus two. It was an unintentional cut-down workout, a virtuoso performance of controlled movement. They also bent over, but that hard part of the day's practice ended for everyone with a lot of weary smiles.

We started them on their cool-down. Circling around a trail and heading into the Woods Loop under glum skies, two of the guys jogged together, with one talking up a storm while the other kept shaking his head.

"No, just be quiet," the head-shaker insisted to the other, "I don't want to hear about that now. Be quiet." The woods swallowed the rest of their argument.

***

You can get some things wrong in a season provided most of it is right. In fact, that would strike many coaches as a typical year, the occasional faux pas forgiven when mixed in with all the rest that counts as normal--or even superlative. And so much the better if the gaffes result from trying too hard. There is a long sports history of excesses in pursuit of excellence being overlooked or condoned as long as they produce public accomplishments someone can brag about. It's the errors of omission, those things left undone, that are usually the most consequential, even if unnoticed outside the team.

The runners pushed our Monday and Tuesday practices hard. League competitions had faded in the rearview mirror. The focus had narrowed to our remaining invitational and then the championship races. It was go-time. But on Wednesday, Mindy was missing again for one of her "appointments." The mother had stopped notifying me. We had a Team Meeting planned that day where the boys' and girls' runners would gather without coaches to privately discuss issues, concerns or requests. A designated meeting leader would report the anonymous results back to Coach G. and I before leaving for the day.

Before the girls could walk off to their meeting site, though, I pulled them aside. Coach and I were frustrated and perplexed. I told them about our observed lack of team cohesiveness—and that we wanted them to consider how to work better together. They stared back blankly, but after a long moment, Sandy spoke. "Can I say something?" She understood the reference.

"Of course," I told her, and she then described instances where Mindy had tried to "take over" activities like Team Meetings or to "control" practices by leading workout efforts. Some of the girls simply stood with blank faces, but others nodded. I glanced around the group and reminded them Mindy had, in fact, been a leader as one of the few to run the targeted summer mileage. I also reminded them of how hard she had worked in practices and how hard she raced. No one disagreed, so I told them that personality conflicts happen, but it's important to work them out. That's what good teams do. They agreed to that too, and Sandy admitted they had not brought it up before, hoping any issues would resolve themselves. "Alright," I said, and told them they were going to delay their meeting to the next day for exactly that reason. I had missed the more important point of their complaints.

It was convenient to dismiss those kinds of problems as get-along issues, something common on scholastic teams composed of teenagers. Indirectly, though, they were telling me it was something else, something more important than squabbles. Years earlier, and on a different team, a talented newcomer had been allowed by administrative decree, to miss half a practice twice a week for music lessons. It was not until months after the season, following an Indoor Track practice where the other top runners chatted with me before heading home, that the subject came up. Every one of the girls in the group said they resented the compromised commitment granted that runner. Rather than invoke team rules that would have pulled Mindy from meets due to absences, rather than ignite another heated confrontation with the parent, I had decided to let Mindy's qualified commitment run its course for what remained of the season. Doing that, I violated a basic trust, the trust other team members had in not only the rules but in my duty to uniformly enforce them. I had let the team down.

***

On Thursday, the teams gathered in our familiar place, and after attendance and after the girls headed toward their meeting spot, Mindy lingered. She said she wanted to talk to me privately. As the girls walked off, some glancing back over their shoulders, Mindy started declaring. A team member had filled her in on the previous day's conversation, and she proceeded to accuse me of manipulating the girls against her, and at the same time defended her right to choose other activities that were "just as important" as team practices. I reminded her of the basic attendance rules. She countered that I allowed others to miss practices, and I had to explain why Tammi the previous season had needed to attend counselling sessions weekly. I suggested we join the girls, allow her and other team members to share their concerns and try to work any issues out.

Mindy shook her head no. In an exasperated tone, she declared she couldn't take it anymore. She said she was quitting the team, reached to grab her bag and then turned to leave. "Mindy," I said, "Let's just meet and work this out." But the words bounced off her back. She disappeared into the parking lot out front and was gone.

I returned to the other girls and told them about Mindy's decision. None appeared surprised or particularly upset. During the argument, I had sensed the confrontation had been deliberate and scripted, the outcome predetermined. The girls had probably known what was coming too. After practice, I e-mailed a summary of the meeting to the AD. There was no reaction from him when he received the mother's angry email that evening charging I had set team members against Mindy. He had probably expected as much.

Coach Vigil had always had it right. His three basic expectations for team success--show up; give good efforts; be a good teammate— were mutually dependent and all of them were required. You couldn't be a good teammate if you didn't show up. You couldn't give good efforts if they weren't ultimately in service to the team and teammates. Any resentment, any distancing by the girls, had nothing to do with anyone's manipulation. The girls were simply affirming Vigil's expectations. Still, they had lost another key runner.

Friday afternoon, one member smaller, both teams boarded our bus for the long ride south to the Newark Valley Invitational. We were late in leaving and took a chance, following back roads once off Interstate 81 at Lisle so we might cut some time. Besides the rolling cinema of hills aflame with fall foliage against a cloud-spotted sky, my shortcut was a bad choice. I kept glancing around every corner, hoping to spot the high school while checking my watch. Finally, we pulled in, and the teams scrambled. The girls' race was first, and they barely had time to drop bags at the team tent site and complete a quick warm-up before reporting to the line. They pinned on bib numbers and starred into the afternoon sun sinking toward a distant ridge. With the gun, they shot off, and I hustled to an intersection on the low flats to watch them power up and down on the course's step hill rising behind the school. Pam was having one of those days; she was going for it, and she finished on the podium with a medal hung from her neck. Erin ran an all-time personal record. "I think that was one of my best races so far," she would declare in her Race Analysis the next day. And she was right. She had mastered the course by measuring her efforts.

The boys also came on strong. Matt finished second individually and Peter clocked one of the top state freshman 5k times of the season. Justin was later emphatic about his effort. "This race was my best race ever for my whole cross-country career." A 30 second personal record was the proof.

Something else, though, dominated the day. As the girls' competitors powered toward the finish astride the track, I had waited. Wendy was still out there, struggling. Not feeling a hundred percent because of a breathing issue, she had nevertheless put everything into her race. Well off her typical finish, she finally pushed across the line and into the runner's paddock, exhausted and leaning for breath. I walked to the end of exit chute from the paddock where other coaches waited for their athletes. She had sacrificed to be the team's important fifth scorer and certainly deserved a pat on the back for that. Suddenly, though, her mother charged out of the crowd, stormed by me and others and into that restricted area. Lifting Wendy, she began guiding her toward the exit as perplexed spectators simply watched. Hand around her daughter, she looked up and saw me waiting. "She's done with this," she said, glaring at me. Taken aback, I said nothing. Passing me, she spit out, "The team mood stinks," and then stalked off with Wendy.

"What the heck?" Coach G. said once I found him and related what happened. Wendy's teammates were also mystified, but reminded they me that she was the team member closest to Mindy. I sent them out to look for her while I attended to the boy's race, but Wendy and her mother were nowhere to be found. When the girls were later called to receive their first-place plaque, the team picture was taken without her.

Back home that evening, I emailed Wendy, telling her the girls' team victory had only been possible because of her gutsy effort and hoping she quickly returned to full health so she could enjoy the rest of the season. She e-mailed back, explaining the problem was not her health but her relationships on the team. That, she wrote, was what was leading her to quit, an assertion I found strange because the other

[300]

girls got along well with her, and respected her efforts. Coach and I both suspected she had been steered toward her conclusion.

Whatever the cause, the result was the same. The girls had lost two top runners in two days. For the remainder of the season, basically a new girls' team would arrive for practice each afternoon, and it would in no way resemble what we had imagined back in June. With subtracted talent, they could not expect to be as competitive, but they would at least be spared additional drama. They could train united, and they could depend on each other. They would finally have the chance to be a Coach Vigil team.

Mike

The first egg landed wide of the mark, but the merry pranksters quickly found their range and soon a fusillade was pelting the high school band members who were marching their routines under evening lights on the high school practice field. Hidden in half-dark behind a fence, Mike and his accomplice quietly hooted in delight as they quickly reloaded and fired again.

The next day, three weeks before our cross-country championship and at the order of a smirking Athletic Director who could enjoy the humor of the moment, they sat with me in the coaches' locker room while I dismissed them from the team. Both sported the obligatory remorseful facades, probably hoping for a mercifully short verbal tongue lashing. And I could have quickly delivered the essentials: 1. That as two of our best runners, they had just screwed the team out of a decent championship effort; 2. At our school you never, ever, mess with the band. Instead, I droned on about putting team before self, about thinking before acting—all the stuff that travels quickly ear to ear when under the age of 18. The next day they handed in uniforms and went their way.

I'm not sure Mike was all that saddened by his shortened season. Built for the track, the long reaches of 5k racing always failed to stoke his enthusiasm. Most cross-country practice days, it was more torture than training. Put him on a track with twelve interval 400's on the agenda, Mike was fine. "He was so tough," Coach Delsole remembered him later, "you could beat him with a stick, and he'd still run 54's all day long."

The trails were another story. Back—and outwardly chastened—for his senior cross-country season, Mike dutifully labored through the harrier training he accepted as the necessary preparation for his more preferred track escapades. At an invitational in nearby Auburn, Mike gave it his best shot and muscled to a top-10 finish in a competitive field. I had a remark handy after his race, thoughts to the effect of how a 4:23 miler can struggle so with a 5k. But I didn't use it. No sense. That day I simply walked up as he came out of the finish chute, gave him a pat on the back and asked, "How'd you feel on that one?"

Mike bent over, took a deep breath, then straightened. "Coach," he said with a sly smile, "it's sooo far."

***

Possibly buoyed by her impressive performance at the Newark Invitational, Pam emailed me the Sunday after: *Do you think that it is too late to reach states at this point in the season?*

I e-mailed back. Pam, *To be blunt, you'd be crazy not to try. There is absolutely nothing to lose and everything to gain. Each year, someone comes out of nowhere to race really well at sectionals. Why shouldn't that be you? And sectionals is still a month--and four weeks of training--away. Go for it. Coach V.*

***

I was standing in the rain with the Baldwinsville coach as we waited for our SCAC Championship coaches' meeting. Jason had again graciously offered his home course to stage that race. The previous year had also been a muddy and wet highlight in that memory of rains. "Jason," I said, joking, "you keep serving up these days, and we'll have to find another site." Jason just shrugged and smiled, drops dripping from the visor of his ball cap. "Hey, then you can take it," he said, only half in jest.

On cue, just before boarding the team bus back at school, the rain had arrived. "It's started," I warned the runners waiting in the hallway to board. "And it's only going to get worse." Puddles had formed and deepened in the parking lot by the time we left, and the rainfall had intensified by the time we arrived at the race site. The middle school gym astride the course was opened for teams, but I knew that would quickly become a damp, noisy and muddy mess, so we claimed a covered entrance alcove on the east side of the building, snugged ourselves in, and never even pulled the team tent from its carry bag. The boy's varsity squad headed out on their warm-up while others pinned all the bib and hip numbers. Two factors were keeping conditions from immediately dipping into the grim range. The gusty early morning winds had abated, and temperatures remained in the mid to upper fifties. Nobody was going to go hypothermic. Soaked, surely, but nothing worse. Forty-five minutes later, the boy's varsity squad lined up on the start line, then tensed as the official blew his alert whistle and slowly raised the start gun.

Most of them had raced so hard and so well the previous Friday at Newark Valley that a mental or physical letdown was possible. A colleague, sports physiologist Russ Ebetts, who has coached on both the scholastic and college level, preaches the "ten-day rule." That is the time a runner's nervous system requires to fully 're-set' from a very strenuous physical effort. The useful rule, though, makes a mockery of your average scholastic race schedule, where Wednesday league meets every week for at least half the season are often followed by important Saturday invitationals. It can be a synaptic overload. But year after year, we pretend runners are soccer or baseball players, and they crank out too many 5k's. Late-season fatigue for some runners comes as no surprise. So here our runners were, on short(but not uncommon) recovery from a hilly and hard Friday race, embracing the mud and rain again.

Find your race early, coaches advise runners, match up to the competitors you expect to be battling in the late reaches of the race with a Goldilocks start--not too fast, not too slow, just right. Neophytes, of course, struggle with the concept because they typically don't yet know the capabilities of their running body and mind. Pacing 'just right' for the majority of the race takes experience, and it requires faith in one's training.

Matt had been searching that sweet spot for several years, and though it was disconcerting to watch a talented runner often go out too hard only to falter in the late-going, I preferred trusting runners to figure that out. That exuberant desire of Matt's to take out the race hard always left him with two options. Either he could, on faith, agreed to control his initial pacing, our we could be patient and provide the training that allows physical and mental fitness to catch up with desire. "Every event is an event of extension," wrote the great Italian coach, Renato Canova about the athlete's efforts to extend endurance at a desired pace. Matt was just about there. He went out behind a crowd of strong runners but maintained a strategic and disciplined pace in the mud so that when the strong F-M trio exerted themselves beyond the halfway mark, Matt went with them even as others faltered and fell back. He muscled his way to 4th, only five seconds out of second place and almost twenty seconds ahead of the 5th place runner. It was his best SCAC Championship finish.

Around the sloppy loops of the course, Peter was in a different place, a freshman confronting the demands of the sport at a high level while simultaneously discovering he had the ability and the drive to meet those demands. But the season had been longer than anything he had previously tackled in the modified ranks, so he was reaching places he had never been before. A soaked, mud-ladened championship race in October was one of those places. Admirably, he raced only seconds slower than his seasonal best, but the veterans surrounding him raced faster, and he finished 15th. The rest of the team's scoring top-5 trailed even further back, with several simply not tackling the conditions forcefully enough. The team placed only 5th in their league division, though they held that place in the 14-team total league merge.

It is entirely possible—and often common—to imagine too much at the same time you are observing too little. Some call that hope, and hope certainly has its place for all coaches standing trailside shouting and exhorting. But that exercise is still just the revelation of what you want, not necessarily what is. If there had been any relief for the girls to at last be freed of team drama and united with a better common commitment, the competitive impact of their recent team losses was readily apparent. On the rain-riven trails, Pam was now their leader, but Pam was still cautious and unable to crack the top-20. The others gave it their best efforts, yet with Carrie, now a potential top-5 team runners, still out with injury, they were simply over-matched and finished 5th. They stood in rain beyond the finish paddock and hugged each other.

Other sections and leagues have their customs, but ours is that all girls' runners are allowed to race the league championship, and the boys get to compete in a separate JV race. That way no team member, the ones who will never qualify for our 10-runner Sectional Championship rosters, ever graduates without at least one opportunity to race a championship. Time standards have been argued for years, but since the girls' numbers are usually smaller and since the boys JV race is placed last, nothing comes of those discussions. Everyone races at leagues.

And that's how Jeremy got where he was. He turned the last corner of his final championship as a Wildcat, and in the pounding rain he began the long upward slant toward the finish. It wasn't the ending he'd envisioned. No gear-grinding push, with crowds lining the chute area to cheer him on. No personal record was in the offing as a culminating grand prize. He was one of the last to finish that day, and most everyone but the timing crew and two or three stalwart spectators had left, making the place a lonely sight. Jeremy lumbered his way up the slant, hair matted down by the rain, singlet soaked and sticking to him. He splashed through a shallow pond that had appeared ten meters out, crossed the finish line and just stopped. The rain washed over him as his chest heaved and he starred outward, as though considering something further off but not discernable to anyone else. His teammates, though, waited at the end of the finish chute, some with fists pumped into the pouring rain.

***

Another day drab with dirty clouds had begun to break open. Distant shafts of afternoon sunlight were poking through onto the hills to our west, and beyond that, just visible on the distant horizon, open sky marked the surrender of the nor'easter that had drenched us for most of the week. Maybe our Marathon Invitational the next day, our last full-team race of the season, would be favored with sunshine. We hoped. Pam was standing with others under our protective overhang and pointing out some of the course details on the Marathon trail map I had taped to the side of the building. The new runners who had never ventured onto the long slants and sharp, short hills of Marathon eyed the map intently. The team had gathered around her in a semi-circle, waiting for my typical 'trail talk' about the course.

The rain had dwindled to nearly nothing. "Pam," I announced, "why don't you do trail-talk for us?" Surprised, pleased and apprehensive all at once, she began and immediately hesitated to find the right word for that long slant down the back field start of the Appleby Elementary School 5k circuit. So of course, others began hooting and haranguing, and then Pam was flushed and embarrassed, just making things worse. I interrupted and reminded them how to listen and ask appropriate questions, then gave Pam some help with the descriptive walk-through. It never fails; they crave the spotlight and the attention until you actually give it to them. The session ended with some others contributing comments from past experience-- the gradual ups that deceptively wear on you, other places where you might catch a short recovery, and others still where you hoped there would be no shoe-sucking mud. Heads of the veterans nodded when I warned them again about being "suckered out too fast" on that opening downhill, but a lot of the first-timers just starred and strained to absorb all the information they would match to the actual topography in less than twenty-four hours.

"O.K.," I said, wrapping up, "you know what comes next." All eyes trained in on me. "The dreaded pre-race timed run." Everyone knew my distain for most timed runs, a conviction which perfectly opposed theirs.

"Oh no!" one of the runners feigned, "please, no."

"Oh god!" chimed in another, "don't make us do that."

Then came a cacophony of voices in briar patch fashion, pleading for something else, anything else, all of it mixed with smiles and laughter. My only demand was the insertion of several up-pace minutes, just to cover all the energy systems. As they grouped and headed onto the deserted training trails, sunlight bullied its way through the clouds.

Down I-81 south of Cortland, as it contoured hills above the Tioughnioga River, we rounded a corner and confronted a dense bank of morning fog. It filled the valley below like cotton puffs stuffed in a bowl. Poking above the fog, the surrounding hills paraded their quilt colors of mid-autumn, colorful forests interspersed with still-green fields. I directed the bus driver down the exit ramp. We descended into the fog and through the hunched buildings of Marathon where a signature sculpture reared in front of the Three Bear Inn. The driver turned left, back under the interstate, took another left at the cemetery, and then we climbed Albro Road to Appleby Elementary, the site of the Marathon 5k racecourse.

Figures shuffled by in the dense mist as we unloaded. Our group tramped the team tent through the wet grass and set up along one sheltered wing of the building. A gun sounded in the watery silence, and the first Modified race of the day was off, though we couldn't see it. We knew our boys and girls modified teams, who had left at 6:15 a.m., were uphill somewhere, readying for their races that came next. But unless the fog suddenly lifted, there wouldn't be much race to watch.

Our tent crew quickly completed their job while others pinned and organized bib numbers. Coach Gangemi and I started around the school track to try and spy what we could of our boys modified start. A coach hurriedly jogged by, towing a delinquent young charge and urging, "Hurry up! You only have four minutes." Coach G. glanced at his watch "Actually, three," he said, shaking his head. "That dude's not going to make it." Minutes later, a start gun popped in the mist, and we caught a shrouded glimpse of the boys large schools modified runners charging down the long slant, their race day already on full throttle. Virtually unseen, our Modified boys earned a strong second-place finish, but just as the girls modified race lined up, the fog began to dissipate, and we could watch most of Claire's start-to-finish out-in-front individual race victory. Her teammates placed six runners in the top-20 to take the title.

The emerging view was vintage Marathon Invitational. Perched high above the town and river valley, the school grounds and its racecourse only grudgingly yields snips of level terrain, much of that engineered for level playing fields. Most of the place—and the course--is on a tilt. Racers spend a lot of their time gradually going up, or gradually coming down. Throw in a few short, steep rises plus twists and turns of the lower trails, and the course can only be graded as tough. Not many racers arrive expecting anything better than a course PR. A wet, muddy day elevates everything to a whole other level of demanding. And so, of course, a lot of runners just love the place and tell their 'war stories' to prove it. A late-season Marathon contest, fair weather or foul, imprints itself in the minds of coaches also. I was on our 17th trip there—and greeted a lot of familiar faces.

Coach and I trudged up to the start line for our boys unseeded varsity race. Because of past successes, the meet director had awarded us berths in both the unseeded and seeded varsity races. But we were smaller that season and with two top runners were away taking PSAT's, we had to move others up, leaving only six in the seeded race and the minimum of five in both the unseeded and JV contests. If anyone went down or dropped from those two races, the team would finish incomplete. We were cutting it close.

As the unseeded squad of five surged out on warm-up strides, Steve shuffled up. Due to line up for the varsity race, he simply looked awful, with shoulders slumped and long, drawn eyes. Without telling me, he had roused himself from bed, sick, then curled in a bus back seat all the way to the race course. He attempted his warm-up, but basically he was just proving he could not possibly compete—and he proved himself right. He stood there, the picture of dejection. I just gave him a pat on the shoulder. "Steve, if you have a ride here, you should just get yourself home." Head down, he nodded. "Feel better," I said as he hobbled off, creating a third group with absolutely no margin for error.

The sun was doing its work, though, and it would just be a matter of time before the dissipating fog gave us back all the course and the valley vistas beyond. In short order, the start official fired the unseeded teams off the line. They charged down the slant, slowly closing ranks. As warned, our runners resisted the urge to blast the opening descent. They settled into their paces and as a team finished mid-pack with strong races. Despite the difficulty of the course, four of the five ran seasonal PR's. Trent's was by an impressive twenty seconds, while Justin blasted the second fastest 5k that had ever passed beneath his feet.

The faint shouts and cheers of fans at the unseeded race finish drifted up as the boys seeded teams—ours included--found their start boxes and began final preparations. I watched our guys stride out partway down the slant, pull up and gather, then turn and jog back toward me. They were without Aidan, our important #3 runner, who was probably hunched over a hard question at his PSAT's. They were without mercurial Jack, who on any given day could either disappear into the JV ranks or excite everyone with a team top-7 race. And they were now without Steve, headed home sick. After delivering start instructions on his megaphone, the starter called the countdown: five minutes; three minutes—no more runouts; one minute. Coaches backed off and racers stepped to their ready positions two steps behind the start line. Then the starter's gun tilted skyward as runners stepped forward and crouched with intent stares. With the bark of the blank shell, they charged off.

Matt made up his mind early. Down the start slant, into and around a small grove of trees and then right back up to cross in front of the start line before descending again, he led the field with a small gap on a chase pack of other runners, including a talented Watkins Glen competitor. Matt had done his homework and understood that runner would be his race. Standing trailside, I shouted encouragement. Only a few competitors back came Peter, already off to a strong start, aiming for a podium top-6 finish. The main body of runners streamed past, and suddenly there was neophyte Andy as our #3, racing the best 5k of his short career. Tom and Ryan were engulfed further back in the main column of runners. I shouted at them to move up.

Down through the lower trails, circling back around the finish and then alongside the track, Matt was locked into his race with his Watkins Glen competitor. By the time he climbed the course and circled around behind the start line a last time, he had lost the lead. His adversary was powering down the slant with only a half mile remaining. Matt was in danger of being gapped and losing contact. "This is it, Matt!" I yelled. "You have it in you. Go!" They disappeared into the lower trails, and I turned to wait for the others to pass.

At Marathon, our races typically come quickly, one after the other. Since I take start-line duties while Coach G. handles the finish, I rarely get to see the ends of races. Fabulous finishes are always stories told to me later by Coach G. or the runners themselves. But this day, I had a little time before the final boys JV competition, so I jogged down toward the finish paddock. I didn't make it in time. Our boy's seeded team, their day's efforts complete, was still sitting, removing timing chips and munching apples in bright sunshine. I found Andy and offered congratulations. He had just clocked his third straight 5k PR, this one by almost thirty seconds. Our critical fifth team runner, Ryan, had pushed himself, despite sore shins, and

Tom, our number four, came in only a few seconds off his seasonal best. They performed well, despite missing critical runners.

Peter was smiling when I found him. "What place?" I asked, knowing he had been battling for a spot on the podium. He smugly held up six fingers. "I was a little behind in the trails, but I said, 'no way' and went." Later, he received the fastest freshman award for boys.

Matt, meanwhile, sat nearby, lacing his shoes with tired satisfaction. He caught my eye and flipped over his place card to reveal a #1. "But you were almost ten meters back going into the trees," I said. He simply nodded. "What about coming out?" I asked.

That's when Matt smiled. "About ten meters ahead."

"So you raced the corners, didn't you?"

"Yeah. Hard."

Theirs was not a win, only 5th place, but it was a great group effort. The girls later added a top-5 finish of their own. Half of them ran seasonal PR's on the tough slants and hills of Marathon. They performed too.

[314]

Shawn

The officials pulled him off the looped course at the two-mile mark of the McQuaid Invitational. They were enforcing the new Straggler Rule that I had stupidly missed in the fine print, a procedure intended to keep slow competitors from being overtaken by fast front-runners in the next race, a circumstance guaranteed to make a mess of the meet scoring. It was just as well I wasn't there, that his mother was the one who saw him welling up with shock and disappointment. To me, he always seemed too massive for anything like that, more a linebacker who laced up running flats every afternoon than a distance runner.

The next fall, Shawn gave up his junior year of cross-country to prepare for a shot at winter's basketball team. When that didn't work out, he was back for his senior season as a harrier, still huge by runner standards. McQuaid and its Straggler Rule was first on his agenda. I offered to allow him to sit it out and avoid the rule, but he would have no part of that.

It wasn't even close. He sailed by the officials sharpening their hooks for the slower runners behind him. Next, he homed in on the 26:00 5k that had eluded him for years. That proved more vexing than outrunning the Straggler Rule. The remaining October efforts—27:34.0, 26:27.2, 26:31.4—slipped by like lost starlings. Time was running out, but he caught a break at our league championship, his final race as a Wildcat. Hills were replaced by rises. The footing was decent. He'd have momentum in his favor, and heart was never the issue.

There were other memorable team moments that season, but what sticks in the mind's eye are the low, dappled autumn hills surrounding the championship course, the wisp of a comfortable breeze and big Shawn in the middle of it all: *Shawn out strong, holding his own at the back of JV pack. Shawn pushing the middle mile, growing in confidence while team members and family grow in anticipation. Shawn in the race's late stages, suddenly understanding it's there for the taking and digging deeper. Then a teammate is bolting across the closing loop, screaming at him "You can do it Shawn! You can do it! Keep driving!" And Shawn's doing just that— charging for all he's worth around the last turn, a tractor-trailer on a race course with Peugeots, taking mark on his final finish line as the crowd's cacophony matches those pumping arms and massive churning legs.*

Into the chute, Shawn wobbled with an exhausted smile. Overhead the clock read: 25:56.8.

And we have the photograph to prove it.

***

It was a lot to ask of Carrie. All September, she had been industriously toiling along, adding her focused effort to those of her teammates and with no top-runner expectations beyond, perhaps, making the ten-person sectional squad. She had never been a scorer for the team, but then, after returning from several missed competitions due to a minor injury, suddenly she found herself a team top-5 runner, promoted by attrition into a critical role. Carrie was a hurdler at heart, a diligent one at that. Her parents actually bought her a hurdle, and it came out of the garage in the off-season whenever the weather permitted. Carrie agreed to cross-country to build toughness and speed-endurance for the four hundred intermediate hurdles event and because she liked her potential teammates. She was typically reserved and cooperative; a stifled giggle amounted to one of her more emotive efforts. Carrie, though, never shied from the work. After hard efforts on the longer distances, she leaned, wide-eyed, gasping, looking as if she might simply topple over if you pushed her with a finger.

So, in the unstated drama that can happen when something is unexpected, there she was, thrust into an unfamiliar role and awarded the almost impossible mandate to suddenly become something more than what anyone expected her to be only weeks before. Our sport creates those kinds of dilemmas. Once, years earlier, something similar had been the story of the entire season. We'd had four runners on that team who were able to train on comparable levels, a simple validation of individual physiology and genes. Then there were several others, with less talent, who followed further behind. Willpower or preparation were never factors in that wide gap. The gap manifested itself regularly in meets, and dark humor set in as the season progressed. The inevitable four front-scoring runners would come in reasonably close—then we would wait for the necessary fifth, who was usually preceded, in large meets, by 10, 15, as any as 30 runners. We would watch a team score ballooning before our final scoring member lunged across the finish, spent. There was nothing we could do, and there was no one to blame because those inflated team scores were never the fault of our fifth runner, who gave it her all. One meet, I stood with Coach Delsole, watching the process play out yet again. "Oh geeze," I muttered as competitors flew by. "Four runners, then a cup of coffee." Coach laughed.

Carrie never volunteered as a cup of coffee, but that became her role, and she did her level best with it. We knew the gap would exist because we had seen it in the early meets, those before the injury, where her unselfishness and pure work ethic had led to finishes as high as seventh for the team. But the time that now ticked by before she followed teammates across the line was two and a half minutes--on a good day. That's a lot of places. And of course, the urge would be to concoct some unique training partnership or some drill that would magically inject such a runner with heretofore unknown abilities and so close that gap. A forced ah-ha moment. But beyond encouragement and exhortations, we fought that urge. It would not have been realistic--and certainly not fair.

***

The three weeks following our Marathon Invitational before the Section III Championship were clear of meets, with time to just train. And the teams were smaller. Sectional rules allowed us only ten racers for that early November championship, and though we had been diligent about mapping the team depth charts based on late-season efforts and about closely watching practice efforts, there were some bittersweet decisions about who would train on and who would hand in uniforms.

The first Monday of those small-team days, they ran repeat miles on the Woods/Outer Loops of our training trails. It was a sluggish day--and understandable after the races and weather of the previous week. Matt was suffering a slight, nagging muscle strain that kept him from the workout, but the other stubborn guys went after each other with all the zeal they could muster for a Grunt Monday practice. The girls front four all pushed together as though attached with ropes. Then came Carrie.

Tuesday, the runners were shuttled to the Erie Canal. By the time they arrived, the rain was pounding down, and they bounded off the shuttle bus, racing for our covered pavilion, heads and shoulders hunched. When nothing changed after attendance and some training talk, I sent them out into their meteorological fate on a run to Amboy and back. They returned soaked, and there was nothing to do after that but get them home as quickly as possible.

Wednesday, we went to the track. Chrissy was out with a minor injury. Steve was ill and home from school. It was cloudy, but the rain had surrendered, leaving behind just a slight breeze. The agenda was one of their track favorites: 2-2-4 x three sets, with a two-minute recovery between the 200m and 400m efforts and a 3-4 minute recovery between sets. They were run as close as possible to 1500/1600 pace. The runners enjoyed the quickness of the work, and Carrie was happy to see her per/mile gap from the others shrink. Afterward, the two teams sat briefly for meetings. Sandy brought back the girls' sheet and handed it to me while the others headed off the track. Under one category I had suggested for discussion, "Mood of the Team," they wrote down just four words: confident; stronger, more motivation.

Thursday, back on our middle-school training trails, the troops got pretty much what they wanted, a 10-10-10 fartlek, then two strides and two sprints before plyo drills. All the school playing fields lay quiet, deserted. No soccer or football teams were still practicing or competing. Not a soul in sight. Coach G. was away at the winter coaches' meeting. For the first time in twenty-one years, I would not be at that meeting, having retired from Indoor Track and handed over the teams to Coach Palmisano. When the athletes circled for plyo drills, the sun was practicing for the season ahead with an early disappearance behind a low bank of clouds in the west. It seemed a lonely time of the season.

On Friday, they ran a reduced number of hill intervals. At certain points of a season, some training aims more at psychological than physiological benefits--and this was one of those. Matt was back at full strength, so he pulled Peter out to faster circuits, with Aidan not far behind. The rest of the guys, though working hard, were less predictable, but the girls top four again ran thick as thieves, separated most intervals by no more than an arm's length. The season had hardened in the fields, and any leaves still clinging to forest trees were volunteering themselves with every slight wisp of wind, fluttering down. Through them came Carrie, creeping closer still.

We could never have imagined anything better—or wished to. Ours was a Monday mid-Fall gift, an afternoon of sun and golden fields, of harmless clouds and autumnal stillness. The Sectional Championship was still two weeks off, but drawing closer. I told the team members that the previous training week had been good, very good. I did not tell them those days had been the sense of unity they'd lacked much of the season, but Coach and I were thinking that. The productive and purposeful work of those afternoons, wet or dry, had simply driven home the point that common goals and mutual sacrifices are the foundation of successful and worthwhile teams. Talent can't cheat on that.

The teams walked out to the back field and dropped water bottles at the upper entrance to the Inner Loop. They were after 6 x 800m on the sinuous loop. Just over four months earlier, in late June's long light, twelve Wildcats had assembled for a voluntary summer run at this same spot for that same work--and the entire team had run that same practice just the month before. So, the workout had a seasonal history, a circular sense to it, though I could just as easily have imagined some great runners of our past blasting down the final slant to a finish cone and bending for air, exhausted and proud at the same time.

I stated the day's intent: *Go at your weakness by using your strengths. Push back at the pain and see what that gets you.* More discretely, I told Peter to try and shrink the distance to Matt, and to Carrie I just said keep up the good work.

Grouped, they charged out, disappearing up the curving rise and reappearing only after walking back from the finish cone area hidden by birches to report and record their times. I had a copy of that previous workout that I slipped onto the clipboard for the sake of curiosity. On their opening interval, Matt and Peter ran almost thirty seconds faster than their first one of the previous month. For Pam, the improvement was less, but still over ten seconds faster. Everyone got in on the act because the signal had been sent: good start; keep it going. The four girls tightened as a group and came in strong on #2, seven seconds ahead of their previous. They didn't know the numbers I surveyed surreptitiously, but they certainly heard me congratulating them, and they saw me smiling. On #3, they went thirteen seconds quicker. Then came the hard intervals, four and five, where their numbers ballooned slightly, but were still impressive improvements. For them, anything under 3:10 on the twisty loop was solid, on-pace work that would either maintain or advance fitness. Coach and I watched them queue for #6, their final effort. "Come on," I urged, clapping, "let's dig deep." They surged out and vanished up the rise. I walked into the field, hoping for a photo of the girls group coursing the trail but caught only a fleeting glimpse of the four slanting down toward the finish cone and into the birch grove that hid them. I heard tired whoops, and when I thrashed my way back to the start area, they were smiling and tiredly sipping from their water bottles. "Well?" I asked.

"2:58," Pam said, grinning.

Their second practice week would end in November, month six of the season, so the weather gods probably thought, *what the hell*, and delivered a second afternoon of late October sunshine, warmth and stillness. Following their Monday push, no one complained about some easier Tuesday running on the trails. I had meandered that day, spotting them here and there enjoying the charitable temperatures. A group of girls emerged from the Woods Loop, approaching Three Corners just as a farmer's combine churned a corner of the leased Ike Dixon Field, gathering the season's grain. By Thursday, though, our luck ran out. It was Halloween, and I was back under the protective metal canopy of the Erie Canal pavilion, waiting for the shuttle bus and listening to a percussive rain symphony on the roof above. Things looked grim for the trick-or-treaters later, and my second-guessing began. I should have run an indoor workout on the middle school oval. I should have just cancelled and given them what they hadn't enjoyed all season—a serendipitous day off. But it was too late for either. The athletes were soon racing toward the pavilion, wobbling with their heavy bags through the maze of swelling towpath puddles.

Years ago, Edward Deci and Richard Ryan published a paper with the dense title, "Self-Determination Theory and the Facilitation of Intrinsic Motivation." They concluded that motivation which endures (the important clarification) comes from satisfying three basic needs: competency; autonomy; relatedness. They described competency as having a sense of control over the outcomes of one's efforts and the ability to make progress over time. Autonomy meant acting in accord with one's core values and beliefs--in other words, doing something that makes you feel authentic and comfortable with your efforts. Relatedness was simply fulfilling a need to connect with something larger than just yourself.

The runners huddled as I talked about this thing or that. All of them, save one or two, had only a single big push remaining, one all-out race effort ahead in little more than a week. Then they would move on, most eventually appreciating the memories of tough workouts under blue-sky sunlight or hammering rain more than any race--although it was racing that made all the rest possible. Steve Magness wrote: "Doing hard things brings value." Hard had been part of their lives since late August, with a little more left.

Then, suddenly, the rain slackened. The sky lightened slightly. The drumbeat of rain on metal roof dwindled, and ours became just another afternoon like so many others of those spectacularly normal days. They listened as I plotted out their afternoon's work.

November

***

It doesn't matter the time of year or the fact that any modern track can claim the descriptor "all-weather." Tracks are all constructed with one image in mind: situated under warm sunshine and populated by athletes in shorts and T-shirts. That's what we think of when the word comes up. But we had, instead, cold and raw on a Friday track, a day draped by an upper tapestry of dirty clouds. Ryan had apparently missed the weather memo. In a T-shirt, windbreaker, and shorts, he had jogged halfway out to the start line in the 42° breeze as I entered the stadium, then hurriedly passed me going back, mumbling "getting my pants." Welcome to the November, I thought.

Peter strolled in a few minutes later, noticing the three cones placed in ten-meter increments back from the start line. "Step-ups, huh?"

"Yup," I answered.

We had a track day to end our good practice week. At first, I paid little attention to our three dawdlers, expecting them momentarily. The rest of the crew assembled at the track finish line for instructions, then set out on a mile warm-up. On their third lap around, when Erin passed, I asked her, "Where are they?" She seemed to shrug and then called back over her shoulder, "I honestly don't know."

As everyone finished their final lap, Sandy and Pam meandered in, dropped their packs near the start-line entrance and jogged toward me. When they got near, Sandy knew to explain. "I lost my cell phone," she said, "and we had to find it."

"So where's Lori?" Lori was the third of the late amigos.

"She went home sick."

I said nothing, and sent them on their warm-up, a fifteen-minute delay that I refused to shorten. It meant they would start the workout by themselves, and Erin would be without her training buddies. Maybe the two of them could join her for Erin's second and third set, then finish theirs alone. I wasn't sure. I diverted my irritation with the day's only silver lining—no rain.

"Step-ups it is," I told the crew after their warm-up and drills, "but just three sets." Several looks of relief greeted me. "But remember, we are looking for power *and* speed. Feel fast and be fast--*and* as relaxed as possible."

They grouped and started. Erin, lacking any partner, simply toed the line and set off about forty meters behind a boys group that included Trent, Tom, Steve, and Andy. At the end of the first set, three step-up 400's later, I pulled her aside as she recovered. "Erin, do you realize you just finished about the same distance behind the guys that you started?" She seemed surprised. When she readied for set two, her tardy training buddies had just launched into their first set, so Erin braced up and leaned on the line with the boys group.

The gloomy afternoon had closed around them, but all the runners powered on. Erin finished her second--and then her third set--only seconds off the boys group. It was her fastest per mile training of the season and noticeably faster than her teammates. Bent over, she gulped air and glanced in my direction.

"Yeah," was all I said as she offered a weary smile. I tapped my watch and nodded.

***

"Fall back." The lost hour over the first November weekend meant racing afternoon sunsets. For Monday of our Sectional Championship week, we were gifted a fifty-degree day with sunshine. The runners' agenda included a reduced number of longer interval work, but they would sweat instead of shiver. I asked, "Has anyone heard that phrase, 'The hay's in the barn?'"

Blank stares until Sandy braved the question, "Something about being finished?"

"Bingo. Unless you make states, this work is mostly to stay sharp, mentally and physically." Heads nodded "The most important things you'll do this week is to remain healthy and sleep."

By Wednesday, though, they weren't all healthy. It would be their last afternoon of any harder work, but Pam was hobbled by a slight stiffness in her left ankle, something that she said had come on after Monday's long intervals. She didn't know how it happened but said she had a history of ankle rolls, which was news to Coach G. and me. I told her to monitor the ankle and then described the afternoon's work to the team, which was the return to a confidence-building practice of repeat 400's on the back playing fields. They would record only the total times of their two sets of three 400's, and the directions were simple: "I want you to run the first set fast—and then the second set faster."

Most of them did. The two previous afternoons, we had allowed Andy to attend overlapping basketball tryouts, but our attempts at being 'flexible' proved a bad bargain. He practiced poorly, leaving me wondering about a focused sectionals effort now that he had two sports on his mind. The others, though, gave good efforts, so when I suggested they substitute a light GC trail run for their expected speed work to finish, Erin chirped up, "That's an excellent idea!" and off they went.

On Thursday, they bussed to the Erie Canal for some towpath running. It snowed.

On Friday, we could have gathered for a few cold miles and needless talk, but I emailed them to instead go home after school and enjoy a short GC run and strides in their neighborhoods. They finally got that day off.

***

For most of our area teams, the Sectional Championship is the big meet of the season. Though only a steppingstone for the elite squads who are focused ahead to state or even national championships, the rest of us usually hang our hats on that early November team performance. After sectionals, the majority of athletes, finished for the year, go home with the memories. This culminating affair is also the one day of the season when all the sectional teams gather to contest their separate class races. The timing system, though, can create a total merge of all the teams and individuals. So, for our section, that means sixty-plus teams get to see how they match up racing the same course on the same day. Our school program had always considered a top-10 merge finish as the sign of a decent competitive season. Most years, both boys and girls teams have been able to claim that distinction.

By 7:25 a.m., with all the athletes on a cold bus and the equipment loaded, Coach Gangemi had still not arrived. I sat in my seat, wondering if he'd missed his alarm, then checked my text messages. There it was from the previous night: *Hey Jim, I'm at Upstate right now. Dislocated my patella playing hockey a little over an hour ago. They just completed an X-Ray. Just wanted to let you know early enough that I won't be able to make it sectionals tomorrow so you have enough time to contact Coach P. to see if he could go in my place. Praying there is no tear. I'm so sorry that I can't make it. Please tell the athletes what happened and that I wish them all the best of luck.*

[329]

I announced the coach's sad story to the athletes, and we headed out. Later, as the November farm-fields, humbled by early snow, passed beyond the bus windows, Coach G. texted a photo of his right leg trussed up in a brace. Crutches leaned against the wall nearby.

Our early September ride east down the New York Thruway to the Vernon-Verona-Sherrill Invitational, now our Sectional Championship site, had been warmer, a lot warmer. We arrived this day to a thirty-four-degree cemented landscape. With class races rotated each year in the schedule, this year we took our turn as the early race in the coldest part of the day. Following the plan, the girls set up the team tent while the boys began their pre-race sequence. They returned from a warm-up run declaring what I'd suspected—there were some mushy spots near the start, but half-inch spikes would be a disadvantage on the hardened trails and across gravel stretches of the course. The girls, racing two hours later in slightly warmer weather, would evaluate spike lengths closer to their gun time.

Country-western tunes blared from the stadium speakers, but no one was dancing. Spectators in puffy down jackets and athletes wrapped in blankets shuffled by as boys Class A teams completed their preparations and donned spikes. Clouds had begun sliding in from the west and threatened to subtract a few degrees from the projected high temperature of 38°. At our start-line box, the athletes left layers on during strides and sprints, waiting for the five-minute warning. "You want to go home knowing you've given it your best," I had told them. "That's what you want for your teammates, your best race." A few minutes later, the starter barked, "No more runouts!" and shortly after, his pistol puffed white against the southern woodland hills. They were off.

For most runners on those cold November days, a season spanning six months--and almost half a year--shrinks to its final minutes and seconds. This is their last chance to take chances. Most of the team had gotten out well, had made the efforts to put themselves in the race positions that mattered. They wound in and out of the quiet wooded areas, up and down hills and past crowds roaring support. Coaches and spectators familiar with the course rushed from place to place like a golf crowd. As I shuffled around to spot my passing runners, the entire season was etched on their faces. Looks of determined effort early, evidence of mounting fatigue in the middle stages, late signs of surprising struggles or opportunity—all passed by my shouts and exhortations. Matt had gone out hard with the leaders, faltered mid-race as he fell back into the chase pack, then rallied and began moving up. Peter passed, heading into the woods a final time as I counted the number of competitors not on the expected winning team. That magic number was five. Those first five individuals, after the winning team members were subtracted from results. would also advance to states. Too far back, Peter appeared unlikely to make it, but he was pushing hard and would eventually cement his position as one of the state's most talented freshman runners with fifteenth place, the best 9th grade effort in our section. Aidan, Tom, Ryan—all charged home with nothing left in the tank, having given it their best. Only Andy struggled, finishing out of the team top-7, a promising runner who, for unknown reasons, would eventually promise himself never to run cross-country again. I took a team picture of the weary crew, and then later, just before the girls' race, I ducked inside to the gym to watch Matt smile on the awards stand with his individual medal and knit cap. His late charge had propelled him to sixth place and to the third individual qualifier spot. The boys' team had placed only sixth, a disappointment, but Matt would represent the Wildcats at states.

Back outside, I found the girls at the team tent and in the final stages of preparation for their noon race. They laced up racing flats, secured bib numbers to their singlets, then layered back up before heading to the start line. The temperature had moderated, but only a little. Cold racing was ahead. On the line, several teams beside us had lathered up bare skin with baby oil, a strategy popularized by the dominate Saratoga teams of old. Its scent, slightly reminiscent of sunscreen for the beach, wafted incongruously down the chilly start line. Called to attention by the starter, runners hopped and shuffled in place to stay warm. With the gun, our last team endeavor of the season charged off.

There were no competitive miracles waiting on the cold trails, just the demands of a hard race with teammates. Our runners, none top-20 finishers or challengers for a state championship qualification, were fighting exhaustion by the time they labored up and over the final rise, passing through a funnel of cheering spectators. Down the backside of the rise and into the final loop on the flats below, Pam, Lori, Sandy, and Erin made their last pushes. And that cup of coffee wait after them was the shortest of their incongruous second season. Carrie muscled her way up and over the rise, battling to the fastest 5k of her career. The team's eighth-place Class finish was the team's lowest in twenty-two years, but we didn't care. A less public form of victory mattered more.

Later, back at the team tent, Friends of Wildcats Cross-Country parents had set up tables of post-race snacks. I called the boys together with the good news that they'd placed 10th in the total 66-team sectional merge, an improvement of fourteen places over the previous year. The girls' team finished out of the top-20, but with best efforts. The girls had switched to running flats and they then headed out on a quick cool-down. Only a short distance away, out along the school's back parking lot, they stopped, circled, and draped arms over each other. The chant of their start-line team cheer rose through the chilly air, then they jogged off into the back fields. When they returned, I asked about that. "Oh," Erin explained, "we were rushed at the start line and didn't get a chance. We just wanted to make sure we did it together one last time."

***

The morning after sectionals, Tom, Steve, Aidan and Trent joined Casey for a little unannounced 'recovery day' workout. They ran the Syracuse Half-Marathon.

"We took it at a good conversational pace," Tom emailed me later, "and ran together until mile 10."

I didn't ask what came after that.

Coach Delsole

Seasons ago, we had some runners one afternoon who weren't giving their best. They offered up multiple reasons for why they couldn't run faster, but mostly they were offended about being called out. It reminded me of the story Coach Delsole told once about the women's volleyball team he coached for a couple of years at a local college. In practice one day, some of the women weren't anticipating quickly enough and getting to their correct defensive positions, those spots on the court where they could narrow down the spiking angles of their opponents. Coach was barking at a few of them about reaching those positions faster. Several of the ladies didn't like the attention and insinuated that Coach was demeaning them. So he stopped the practice to explain. "Listen," he told everyone, "if I'm yelling at you to get to a certain position more quickly, that's not personal, that's just about playing better. But if I yell about your position and then tell you your dog's ugly—that's personal."

And then there were three of them. Matt was bound for states, while Peter and Aidan would join him to train for the Nike regional race the three of them would contest the Saturday after Thanksgiving, still almost three weeks away. They would soldier the XC season out to six full months, and I again, in spontaneous moments, would appreciate the stunning breath of the season. Spring-Summer-Fall. Six months in the life of a sixteen-year-old is 1/32nd of his or her life, a significant amount of time for a singular endeavor. That investment commands, whether conscious or intuitive, an appreciation of time passing. Dry-throat heat surrendering to turning leaves and, finally, early snow and cold. Small wonder that, for many runners and coaches, it remains their favorite sport. You don't just complete a cross-country season; you live it.

After his half-marathon 'recovery run' on Sunday, I had e-mailed Aidan to take this workout off. No surprise, he agreed, noting his legs felt "tired." Matt and Peter would forego our training trails and tackle the Monte Vista up-and-around near school, our .4-mile circuit, five times. With me atop the steep initial rise, we were a small crew.

Matt and Peter went at it in the mid-30° degree weather. The target was what it had been for the past month: faster than current 5k race pace. As they completed their fourth interval, an elderly lady, bundled against the chill, walked my way on her upper circle afternoon perambulation and stopped near me. She stared at the two runners hunched over, breathless for a moment before straightening. "Cross-country?" she said, turning to me.

"Yes ma'am," I answered.

She considered the two of them as they jogged slowly down the steep rise. Then she smiled. "All your athletes know Monte Vista well, don't they?"

I nodded. "Yes ma'am, they certainly do."

I turned the antique key in the old-style lock and entered my tastefully appointed Allen Room of the North Hero House, our lodging for the night. Matt and Peter, his "travel buddy" for the state championship, were staying in one of the separate guest houses down near the cold, blue waters of Lake Champlain. Ten years earlier, when the championship was also staged on the SUNY Plattsburgh campus, I had abandoned thoughts of finding any reasonable lodging in the immediate Plattsburgh area and looked further afield. By chance, I found the North Hero House Inn, on North Hero Island in Vermont, a short ferry ride from Plattsburgh. The rates were competitive in their off-season, and a greenhouse off the back of the house had been converted to a restaurant with a lounge area and fireplace. Our three athletes in the championship that year, their small entourage of parents and the bus driver had loved it—so I went back.

I had driven Matt and Peter north through the Adirondacks to Plattsburgh earlier that day. We picked up Matt's bib numbers, and he and Peter jogged a course preview. The week's weather had inflicted damage to the championship course. Brutal mid-week cold had relented enough to allow snow and mud to make a mess of several areas, so the course had been re-routed in three places. Matt and Peter returned after making sense of the new route and described the re-routings. Later, after we left the course to catch the ferry to North Hero Island, re-calculations by meet officials would find the 'new' course longer than a 5k, a state violation, and a fourth re-routing followed. Plummeting temperatures and some snow that night would force still a fifth--and final--re-routing only minutes before Matt's 9:00 a.m. Class A race on Saturday.

Except for some locals, that evening we enjoyed a quiet dinner at the inn's greenhouse restaurant. A fire crackled in the lounge area as Matt described what he was aiming for, the top-20 medal finish that had eluded him at two previous state championships. Re-adjusted course or not, this was his last shot. Before we finished dinner, I spoke with the manager about our planned pre-dawn departure the next morning, and she said she would take care of everything. Passing through the main lobby on their way to an early bedtime, the boys collected their basket of muffins and fruits left for them at the main desk.

***

I pulled the car down to the boys' cottage at 6:15 a.m. The dashboard thermometer read 10°.

"Well, I didn't have a good night," Matt said as he and Peter loaded gear and plopped into the rear seat. I listened to him explain how he'd risen around 2:00 a.m. and thrown up, presumably due to the salmon dinner that did not agree with him. I said nothing except "Oh boy" and we pulled out onto Rt. 2, aiming to make the 6:45 a.m. Cumberland Head--Grand Isle ferry.

About two miles down the darkened island, Peter asked, "Were we supposed to turn in our room key."

"Did you get an old-fashioned room key or just a computer card?" I answered.

"A room key."

Shaking my head, I pulled into a farmer's driveway, turned around and headed back to North Hero House. Peter hustled in, left the key on the room dresser, and we repeated the start of our early morning trudge. Notions of dawn were appearing in the east, beyond the Green Mountains across the lake. We sped by snow-covered farm fields and mostly darkened houses, pulling up to the ferry just in time to load. Bundled boat attendants raised the stern gate and the captain churned us west over dark waters. It was still bitter cold—12 degrees—but with only a slight breeze. Distant Adirondack mountains hunched in a faded pink pre-sunrise. I ventured out on the open deck for a photograph and quickly retreated.

The transit went well, though, and at the race site a parking attendant waved me through to a spot close to the field house where tables inside had been set up to serve as sectional 'tents,' a welcome refuge from the cold. Matt and Peter headed out on Matt's warmup while I chatted with other arriving coaches.

At 8:45 a.m. Matt, Peter and I stood on the start line with officials who were confused about the starting boxes for the different sections. I pulled up the states information on my phone and showed them. Then, as other competitors completed strides and sprints before the 9:00 a.m. start, I walked Matt a short distance out from the start line for a private chat.

"Matt, listen" I told him as he eyed me, "you only have two choices. You can either let your night illness become an excuse for a bad day or you can push that as far back in your mind as possible and just race. You're O.K. now-- and this is states. This is it. Focus on what you want, and you'll be fine." Then I left him and Peter in the last minutes before the gun and trotted to a selected vantage near the upper loop where I could spot him at least three times passing on the course.

Other coaches and spectators with the same idea congregated on the corner of the loop. We heard the faint gun shot in the distance, then shortly saw the runners curving up and around the opening section of the course. Soon, they had circled behind the field house and came charging up and along the walkway toward us. In the mass of churning legs and white breaths, I spotted Matt back somewhere around 30th, not the start he wanted. They circled the short, reconfigured loop around a snow-covered baseball field and came back at us. As he passed and headed into the larger lower loop, I shouted encouragement. He had already picked up a few places.

Then we all waited. Looking around, I noticed course management was lacking. People were standing where the runners would circle back on the upper loop, so I and several coaches mentioned this to an official, who managed to move the crowd back. Long minutes later, the leader re-appeared, and the crowd surged forward again. Matt came through the tight quarters in 28th. "Gotta go Matt!" I screamed. He powered down a utility road, around the ball field in reverse direction and circled back. "Twenty-three! Twenty-three!" I screamed as he barreled by. "Go! Go!" Then I turned to walk back to the Field House, knowing it was another finish I would not see. He wanted that top-20 for a podium medal, and only a huge closing sprint would earn it for him.

Back at the finish line, spent runners, coaches and spectators milled about. Matt was nowhere to be found, but we reunited inside the field house. He had managed to pick off one more runner in the final meters, but placed 22nd, two off the podium. Both chagrined and disappointed, he was still satisfied with his effort. Athletes from the various schools mingled, congratulating each other and swapping war stories about the route and the race. Matt had a personal best for a three-mile reconfigured race distance that would probably never be certified as 3.0, but he would at least have that time for himself. He would know he had shaken off a potential bad day with its built-in excuse, and that he had, instead, gone for it.

After chatting with Matt, Peter and parents, they left for the long drive home. I gathered my things, talked to a few fellow coaches about the course, and then decided to head out myself. The northern route through the cold enclaves of Malone and Potsdam and Canton took me first northwest along Route 190, over the low, northern hills of the Adirondack range and past rugged farm fields, some now sculpted with wind turbines. I wove up and down, through small towns. The snow was deeper there, with the land visibly descending on the right side to become the distant St. Lawrence River plain. I left the radio off and simply watched frozen landscapes pass by. Increased traffic on the clear, wide lanes of Route 3 out of Canton seemed a disappointing intrusion, and all the miles south from Watertown on I-81 were only too familiar. Later, shortly after arriving home, the meet merge came up on Leonetiming. Matt's 43rd place in the day's total of 476 state championship runners had earned him an individual qualification for the NYS Federation Championship the following Saturday. Our school cross-country season marched on.

***

With the season's subtractions, our annual post-season team banquet the Tuesday before Matt's Federation Championship was a smaller affair. The school cafeteria staff had reserved front tables for athletes, and parents found places further back. From the podium, Coach G. gave a short welcome and recognized those parents who had worked diligently to arrange the evening. I followed with a few quick remarks before dinner about how the athletes would only consider it cross-country if it *was* hard, how real success only came to teams with common commitments, and how the legacy of both our teams would be the efforts they made together. The cafeteria staff then directed all to the dinner, and parents chatted over lasagna or chicken while watching their runners up front laughing and having a ball together one last time. After desert, those same athletes cheered wildly as each of the team award winners they had chosen were called forward. Then Erin and Tom walked to the podium for Senior Speeches. Both talked about the lessons of the sport and the season, about sticking together through the tough times, and both wondered how all the years and the seasons had slipped by them so quickly. They said their teammates were like second families. When we started the slide show to end the evening, athletes further back slid up their chairs and crammed together near the front. With each slide of a teammate covered in mud or making a strange face, their hoots and hollers filled the room until there were no more slides and the lights came back on. Coach G. thanked everyone for coming.

***

November, in our northeast region of the country, is the cat's tail twitching. The sudden gripping cold of the state championship weekend just as quickly shifted elsewhere, and thoughts of winter receded as temperatures for the Federations lead-up week climbed into the low to mid-forties—normal. Our trio of guys coursed the training trails all week, accomplishing not too much and not too little, trying to find that delicate 'just right.' On Friday, with Aidan as Matt's 'travel-buddy' this road trip, we left the high school mid-morning, bound for Poughkeepsie's Bowdoin Park and a course preview. The weather for Bowdoin was predicted to almost reach the fifty-degree mark, practically balmy.

"About three hours forty minutes," I told them. We were going down via the Thruway, though Saturday I would travel back alone on Rt. 17, completing a grand loop, as I had done at states. With a quick stop at the Guilderland rest area, we pulled into Bowdoin about 2:35 p.m. The temperature from our high school departure had risen ten degrees. It was brisk, but pleasant enough at 47°. Aidan and Matt set out on their course preview while I claimed Matt's bib numbers, participation sheet and a complimentary water bottle.

The Bowdoin Park course, though not as storied as other great national icons like VanCortlandt or Mt. Sac, still boasts a long and rich history, one decades old. Generations of runners, some of them future Olympians, have battled its demanding trails and hills. The entrance road to the park drops from an escarpment above the Hudson River and curves down to a large protective flat. Park buildings and shelters

[344]

rim the flat, while others perch astride the grass slope that climbs above a small pond. A recent playground halfway down the road dips toward back fields that stretch north. There's an amphitheater below the expansive grass slope that is used for the meet's awards ceremony, but the sense is that the park itself is one large, bowled amphitheater, something naturally meant to highlight the great river beyond which, for centuries, has just been passing by. Around and through and up and down all this wends the 5k Bowdoin trail.

Every sensible coach who has ever brought teams or individuals to compete in the Federation Championship probably gives similar advice: Respect the course as much as the competition. We tell them that the start across the flat and then the rolls going around the new playground and into the back fields are fair enough. Few of us feel any need to hype the infamous mid-race hill, which, to anyone who has jogged or raced it, is glaringly blunt in its declaration. Those other parts, though, are what typically mess with an athlete's race plans. That slow, slanted gravel drive up from the back field—it wants to take out a runner's legs even before he or she hits the big hill, so we remind the runners to be careful what they measure out there. And they are also told that when they cross the pond outlet coming back, that last counterclockwise tracing of the flat's perimeter before the finish might very well feel like forever--so be prepared for forever. I had offered such advice for over two decades. The athletes receiving it change every year, but the course doesn't. So, when Matt and Aidan returned from their preview jog--and before they began strides and sprints near the finishing chute--we stood out in the mid-Fall sunshine, and I described the course again.

[345]

***

"No frost on the windshields," a fellow coach told me in the breakfast area of our hotel the next morning. Jack had been out for a short run earlier and found the temperature reasonable, in the low forties. No state championship early-morning freezer this time around. And Federation Championship mornings are never rushed. The day consists of only two races, the state's best girls teams and individuals at 12:15 p.m. and the same for boys at 1:00 p.m. So, Jack and I enjoyed a leisurely breakfast, knowing the temperature would climb even higher.

Tracey, another sectional colleague, joined us, and we meandered through a host of run-related topics. Both of them, in different ways, are old-school hard drivers, something I had been accused of a few times myself. They share a basic honesty of expectations—and the knowledge and enthusiasm to back those expectations up. They have the teams and individual runners to demonstrate the result of their coaching. As it turns out, though, Jack also buys a lot of things for his runners because no one else will. By his estimation, he told me over breakfast, the total was up to $7000 from his pocket, which includes transportation to meets not funded by the school and training/racing flats and special singlets. "You do what you gotta do," he explained.

After they left, I mulled a cup of coffee and received a text from Matt about leaving for Bowdoin a little earlier. We settled on 10:45 a.m. Later, I sat in a lobby chair, waiting for the two and thinking about that basic desire for personal competitive excellence, the thing that drives so much of coaching. That desire must be qualified with other important attributes and goals, but it is primary and not limited to the team's best runners. Once it's gone—or even once it begins to ebb—that's when you look at the face in the mirror and ask the important question. Desire lives in the future, so once you are no longer excited to fashion the next possible incarnations of your runners, then it's time to hand the clipboard over to someone who is. I was excited about the day ahead. The sun was shining, and the wind was an almost imperceptible 3-4 mph with benign temperatures. As soon as the two stepped off the elevator, and Matt said he had slept well and felt good, I knew a top-30 finish, his personal goal, was in the cards.

When we arrived, Bowdoin Park, quiet and relaxed the previous afternoon, was a moving mass of cars, buses and people. After parking, we walked down the access road and set up in a shelter near the playground. Kids shouted and laughed on the swings and slides while runners passed nearby on their course warm-ups. At intervals, passenger trains whooshed past on the nearby tracks hugging the Hudson, bound for Albany or New York City. People were walking dogs. The concession stand was doing a brisk business in meet t-shirts. Matt and Aidan started off on their warm-up, and I chatted with Matt's parents, who had arrived.

The two runners completed their warmup routine, one natural as breathing, and with a half hour to go, I signaled them off to the start line, almost a half mile away. I trudged in the opposite direction, to a vantage that would allow me to catch him at least four times during the race. As usual, I would be sacrificing the start and probably the finish, but my mid-race glimpses would be more important. He had Aidan for the bookends.

From my spot, I watched kids frolic on the playground and, beyond, a freighter lumbering up the Hudson. I checked my watch, checked it again, and then again until I heard a faint gun shot and knew the race was on. Less than two minutes later, the pace cart

[347]

popped into view below the playground, followed closely by a thick mass of runners. They veered right, squeezed through several trees and headed up past the playground to loop around left and angle down toward the back field. An exact count was impossible, so after spotting Matt, I estimated somewhere between 30 and 35, a decent start. "Go Matt!" I yelled as he whooshed by in a phalanx of runners gunning the short downslope. Turning, I rushed up an embankment and positioned myself alongside the gravel drive out of the back field. The wait was short. The front-runners of the 249 runner field leaders had already circled around and, led by the pace cart, were powering up the slant of the drive. I began a quick count. Matt came through in 32nd, but all I shouted was "Good! Work the hill!" and then he was gone. The more athletic and nimble coaches bounded up the wooded slope above to catch glimpses of the runners on their hill climb, but most of us just waited for them to circle and come down—and we hoped. I had had a very good runner once who went up that hill in good form, then came down later walking, having exhausted herself on the climb. A few minutes later, crowd noise further up the road meant the front-runners were already headed back our way. The cart dipped into sight, with the leaders right behind. I started counting again, thinking this would probably tell the story of his day. "Matt!" I screamed as he passed. "24!" Stumbling down the embankment, I jogged across the grass field below the playground to a spot where they would exit the back field, circle down toward the pond outlet and begin that long reach around the flats. The lead runners had strung out, with the battle for supremacy now splintered into smaller skirmishes between two or three runners fighting for places, those races within the race. The counting was easier, but I caught my breath with the sight of Wildcat gold. "Matt--13!" I yelled as he churned past me toward that last, endless loop. He disappeared down the creek slope.

There are two questions that characterize those most consequential individual moments of distance racing. Always, they confront the

[348]

runner at an inopportune time, the moments when the pain comes calling late in a race, insisting on surrender. The runner must ask again: *Do I really want this?* and, if the first answer is yes, then, *Can I manage it?* Those questions go to the heart of the sport.

There is, of course, the third—and most difficult--question: *Will I give it my full measure?* Late efforts in important races represent the nexus of trust and desire. A lot can happen in a matter of minutes—or seconds--to tilt decisions. Matt still had that long stretch around the lower flat, scant time compared to the breath of a season, but time enough to answer all the questions. I turned and ran toward the finish line, joining a rushing crowd of spectators thinking the same. As I approached the finish paddock, jockeying for a viewing position, the stream of runners was charging over the final rise and gunning toward home. The announcer barked out finisher names and described the sprint battles.

I didn't quite make it. I spotted Matt in the growing mass of tired athletes piling up under the finish tent. Edging around, I caught his eye, and he maneuvered his way over to join other athletes accepting hugs and congratulations from parents and coaches lining the roped off area. I shook his hand. "Well?"

Matt smiled and nodded. "Tenth."

To coach honestly, with knowledge and integrity, means you are going to do your level best to properly deliver athletes to the moments of those questions and then trust they have the answers. And the venues don't matter as much as the answers. The finest coaching moments come when any athlete, in those hard moments of racing, answers yes three times.

"Unbelievable Matt," I sputtered. "Congratulations."

"He was in eleventh when he passed me," Aidan described later as we sat on the lawn stretching up from the amphitheater, watching the awards ceremony. The afternoon was comfortable. A train rumbled by. Matt described how he had picked off two more from where I last saw him before passing Aidan, who was standing just beyond the pond outlet. Then, there was one more move on the long, last loop into the finish. With our twenty-plus years of history with Federation individual and team qualifiers, only one other Wildcat had ever cracked the top-10. As we lounged with the relaxed and festive crowd of spectators, coaches, athletes and parents, the announcer called the top-40 down by groups for medals and photographs. 40 to 31, 30 to 21, then 20 to 11. "And now," the announcer eventually boomed, "your top-10 individual finishers of the 2019 New York State Federation Championship….."

So much of our sport passes in a shallow stream of cliches and platitudes and the everyday shortcuts of description. It is the athletes, some victorious on the big stages but most not, who are left to construct the actual meaning and the value of their own stories about being runners. And consciously or otherwise, everything contributes: the lonely training miles on morning runs, the long bus rides with teammates, the good days and the bad ones too, the abject failures and the surprises in the rain and the mud. The real stories don't belong to the rest of us, the outsiders. They are privately owned.

Matt was announced, which brought polite crowd applause but also hoots from our small contingent of supporters. He marched down to the amphitheater with all his memories. He bowed his head to accept the medal on a blood-red lanyard, and then he came up beaming.

After, I chatted briefly with Matt and family, then watched them trudge up the park road to their cars and the drive home. My own solo route through the Catskills followed valleys and streams. I left the radio off and watched vistas emerge and pass, a motion picture of momentary places. The hillside forests had unburdened themselves of leaves. The isolated pockets of valley fields stood bleached of summer color. Slanted rays of weak afternoon sunlight cast long shadows along those fields, and around one curve, a flock of geese angled over a nearby hill. Soon enough, the runners of indoor track would be launching again into the early dusk of blustery afternoons, cinching up their collars and pulling on gloves.

Winter was coming.

Afterword

The psychologist, Timothy D. Wilson, wrote that people, once they know the outcome of an important event in their lives, tend to construct explanations which make that event seem inevitable. This "hindsight bias" allows us to reshape incidents, interpreting or adding or forgetting actual elements of the story. "That was it all along" is the quiet mantra of those who validate current impressions by magnifying, remembering, or subtracting whatever necessary to create the story they need. It's a neat human trick, instigated by what Daniel Kahneman termed "the lure of hindsight and the illusion of certainty." We like to think we can predict the futures of athletes based on their time with us, but that usually demonstrates nothing more than hubris. It's better not to predict.

Matt, Aidan and Peter traveled back to Bowdoin the Saturday after Thanksgiving for the Nike New York National Qualifier. The top-2 teams would automatically qualify for the National Championship two weeks later in Oregon. Then, the next 5 individual finishers would also qualify. Matt raced 16th overall in the 205-runner field, a strong effort, but he did not gain an individual qualification. Aidan and Peter, gathering the experience they hoped to bring back in future seasons, finished further back. All three followed cross-country with successful indoor track seasons, with Matt earning a place on our State Championship Intersectional Relay. Then Covid wiped out their entire outdoor season. Matt graduated, but Aidan and Peter looked ahead to further running adventures as Wildcats. They still had things to master—and the opportunities.

Erin, as always, took the winter off from running to participate in the annual winter musical. Then, like others, she lost her final spring track season to Covid and graduated, good-naturedly resisting all my attempts to convince her to join her college's running teams. Competitive training and racing had apparently had its place and time.

Wendy might have changed her thinking about teammates because she returned for more seasons and always gave her best efforts in practices and meets.

Following cross-country, the competitive desire seemed to wane for Pam. After a modest indoor track season and a lost Covid outdoor one, she pondered whether to come back to the trails the following Fall. She trained too little over the summer and then contacted me regarding her dilemma. I suspect she anticipated being cajoled into competing, as I had done before. I simply told her I trusted she was mature enough to consider all the alternatives and make the best decision. She decided to look for an after-school job.

Sandy, who always let her actions speak loudest, completed a successful indoor track season, one that included a school record relay, then watched as her last outdoor track season disappeared with the pandemic. She moved on to college to study biology and continue racing competitively on her school's cross-country team. Undoubtedly, she finished some practices and races on all fours.

Following her absence from the cross-country season, Tammi, curiously, returned to run indoor track. Despite the hopes of coaches, however, nothing much came of it. Her competitive event times were far off those of previous track seasons. Perhaps the social comfort of teammates had been, as she honestly described, the primary motivation. That was her last season as a competitive runner.

And Mindy, after stomping off that October afternoon, never joined another track or cross-country roster. Her story vanished with her.

Lori, David, Steve, Carrie, Trent and others, though, would swell the rosters of future running seasons. They found purpose and meaning in their efforts as runners, so their best chapters were yet to be written.

Acknowledgements

Early in my coaching career, I was surrounded by local experts who could have taught me the finest traditions and all the best practices of guiding young middle-distances runners and creating working teams. These were the Section III coaches with multiple cross-country state championships and individual track and field sectional or state championship runners on their resumes. The only problem was they were too busy coaching. I competed against them every season, though, so I was free to watch their behaviors and the behaviors of their athletes, to listen and to absorb their casual comments and the occasional instructive story that I would file away like a mental pack rat. Al Wilson, Rick Nastase, Mike Guzman, George Ball, Jim Goulet, Jack Reed, Bill Aris, Jim Lawton, and Oscar Jenson, the dean of Central New York coaches—these and others all treated me, no charge, to annual master classes in knowing and teaching the skills that make young adults run far and fast.

The book would have remained a discordant arrangement of memories but for the efforts of four who volunteered time and suggestions and recommendations on the evolving manuscript. Russ Ebbets, running coach and author, asked a lot of good questions and offered just as many suggestions that made me think, clarify, and condense. Jack Reed, also an accomplished coach and author, always found and highlighted the prosaic, and in doing so helped me separate the wheat from the chaff. My longtime friend, mountaineering accomplice and former theater director, Bill Morris, egged on the hidden drama in the supposedly ordinary athletic lives of average scholastic athletes. And my sister, Barb Reilly, commented on the book and its characters as an 'outsider,' which was enormously helpful and exactly what I needed.

Years ago, a previous AD, in a tense meeting regarding his non-hiring of the assistant of my choice, assured me that "assistant coaches are a dime a dozen." In my three decades plus of coaching, that assertion has been proven patently false again and again. Greg Gangemi, a 'baseball guy,' came on as my cross-country assistant and was with me during my most turbulent seasons. His intuitive sense of athletes and knack for seeing what I missed always helped keep principles in play rather than just emotions. My longest partnership was with Coach Delsole, an assistant in all three seasons for a number of years—and before that, my head track coach for several seasons. Lou was one of the master coaches, though he might not have considered himself so. His ability to separate the fluff from the fiber of young athletes, his knowledge of what he coached, his objective honesty, his humor, and his unflinching commitment to the best values of the sport made so many of our teams that much better. This book simply would not be what it is without him.

And finally, thanks to my wife, Marsha. The years of dinner gripes about athletes or parents or administrators, the weekends lost to competitions, the nights home late from practices—she made room for it all, sometimes without good reason. Coaching, in that regard, is always a partnership.

About The Author

For over thirty years, Jim Vermeulen has coached scholastic middle-distance runners in the upstate New York school district of West Genesee. As head coach for varsity cross-country, indoor track and outdoor track teams, he has worked with thousands of aspiring athletes and coached hundreds of teams that have included state champions and national All-Americans. He is also the editor of the 1989 book of climbing stories, *Mountain Journeys*, and for the past five years he has been a monthly columnist on high school runners for the NYMilesplit website. Retired from teaching, he continues to coach cross-country and outdoor track teams. He lives in Syracuse, N.Y. with his wife, Marsha.

www.ingramcontent.com/pod-product-compliance
Lightning Source LLC
Chambersburg PA
CBHW070902120626
46546CB00001B/108